A HANDBOOK FOR NURSES

A HANDBOOK FOR NURSES
Common Medical and Surgical Conditions

N. C. WEST S.R.N., R.N.T.
formerly Group Principal Tutor
West Bromwich Group School of Nursing

HODDER AND STOUGHTON
LONDON SYDNEY AUCKLAND TORONTO

ISBN 0 340 18887 1 Paperback
First printed 1967. Reprinted (with corrections) 1969
Second edition 1975. Reprinted 1976, 1980, 1982, 1984
Copyright © 1975 N. C. West

All rights reserved. No part of this publication may be reproduced or transmitted in any form or by any means, electronic or mechanical, including photocopy, recording, or any information storage and retrieval system, without permission in writing from the publisher.

Printed in Great Britain
for Hodder and Stoughton Educational,
a division of Hodder and Stoughton Limited,
by J. W. Arrowsmith Ltd., Bristol

INTRODUCTION

THE AUTHOR OF THIS BOOK is a Sister Tutor of many years' experience in the art of welcoming pupil and student entrants into nursing. She is specially concerned with the awkwardness of those first few days and weeks when the eagerness to come to grips quickly with an understanding of disease and the treatment of the sick is marred by the shyness and the fear of being made to look foolish by questions requiring simple explanations.

Mrs West knows how to allay many of these fears and presents a simple handbook of explanation of some of the common medical and surgical conditions. In addition, pre-examination nerves may be allayed by a quick reference to such a book of definitions and explanations. Finally, Mrs West thinks of the increasing number of married trained nurses who desire to return to hospital work and require a book which will quickly bring them back into the swing of the modern hospital.

A. J. HARDING RAINS

Professor of Surgery,
Charing Cross Hospital Medical School
University of London.

PREFACE

THIS BOOK IS INTENDED for first year student nurses, for pupil nurses, and for nursing auxiliaries. I have also had in mind those who in middle age now wish to take up some form of nursing duty and those trained in the past who now intend to return to hospital work.

My aim has been to explain in simple terms the nature of the common medical and surgical conditions. Where appropriate, the surgical treatment of certain conditions has been given wider scope. The conditions are presented in an alphabetical fashion, but since there are many alternative names, a short index is included to make reference easier.

Routine nursing procedures are *not* included, as all students are taught these in their first few weeks of training, and there are already many books to which she may refer for further details.

My sincere thanks are due to Dr Robert Evans, M.R.C.P., (Senior Consultant, Lecturer to Nurses, and Lecturer in Clinical Medicine, Liverpool University) for his help, suggestions, and the time he has found to read the medical notes, as they were written. Mr A. Abrahams, F.R.C.S. (Consultant Surgeon, and Lecturer to Nurses) also has my sincere gratitude for similar help with the surgical side.

N. C. WEST

West Bromwich Group School of Nursing

My sincere thanks are offered to Dr P. H. Stevens, B.Sc. (Hons.) M.B., Ch.B., M.R.C.S., L.R.C.P. who has found time to read through these additions and revisions and has given me up-to-date advice and suggestions.

N. C. WEST

Perran ar Worthal, Cornwall
October 1974

CONTENTS

	Page
Introduction	v
Preface	vi

	Medical Condition	Surgical Condition
Breathing and Respiration	14, 75	16, 61, 90
Cancer	17	22, 61
Digestion	3, 20, 24, 29, 37, 56, 91	8, 19, 22, 80, 93
Endocrine System	27, 68, 88	88
Heart and Circulation	3, 5, 6, 9, 11, 40, 82	6, 32, 39, 98
Kidneys and Excretion	25, 68, 79, 97	26, 58, 73, 76
Muscles, Bones & Joints	9, 12	1, 2, 9, 21, 34, 43, 64, 78
Nervous System	2, 30, 31, 46, 67, 71, 86	12, 72, 82
Infections and Diseases	20, 24, 48	
Skin	18	

Index	101

A

Abscess
An abscess is a collection of pus in a bag-like cavity of tissue. Pus is a creamy fluid containing dead white blood cells and the live (and dead) bacteria which have caused the infection. An abscess can develop in any organ or part of the body. When present beneath the surface of the skin it is known as a subcutaneous abscess and it may follow a slight puncture injury caused by a splinter, a pin-prick or a cut from glass.

The patient complains of pain in the part, which becomes red, hot and swollen. There may be throbbing, and movement makes the pain worse. The temperature of the patient may rise, and he has a general feeling of being 'off colour' (malaise).

As pus is fluid, the doctor may be able to feel this on examination (palpation) of the swelling. This sign of fluid is known as fluctuation.

Treatment: Once an abscess has formed it should be opened, usually by an incision with a scalpel, so that the pus can escape. Sometimes a small circle of the covering (i.e. skin) is removed so that the drainage of pus is quite free. Any foreign particle such as a splinter is removed with the pus. A specimen of the pus is collected and sent to the bacteriology laboratory in order that the bacteria causing the infection can be identified, and also to find out how sensitive the bacteria are to various antibiotic drugs (sensitivity test).

Frequently the abscess cavity is kept open by a piece of drainage rubber or tubing, in order that drainage may continue until the cavity has been filled in by the healing tissues.

In order that the drainage tube does not disappear into an abscess cavity it is pinned, crosswise, by a sterile safety pin. The drainage tube may need to be moved or shortened regularly every one or two days as ordered by the medical staff. If no drainage tube is inserted, the cavity may be packed lightly with sterile gauze. Should the gauze be too tightly packed it will act as a stopper and prevent the cavity from draining and healing up.

A — A HANDBOOK FOR NURSES

The dressings may need to be changed frequently. Strict aseptic dressing technique (according to the hospital routine) must be observed in order to prevent infection spreading amongst the patients (cross infection).

Acute Rheumatism (see p. 83).

Adenitis

Adentis means inflammation of a gland, and it is a term usually applied to the inflammation of lymph glands (lymph nodes), when it is called lymphadenitis. The cause of lymphadenitis is infection which has been carried by the lymph from a neighbouring part. The glands become large and tender. Glands of neck (cervical lymphadenitis) may thus follow a sore throat, tonsillitis, or from scratching a lice-infested scalp.

In an acute infection the enlarged glands may return to normal after the cause has been successfully treated. Sometimes abscesses may form and require opening (incision). In a chronic infection such as tuberculosis the glands may remain enlarged, and they may become hardened by a deposit of calcium (calcification). If a tuberculous abscess forms the swelling does not feel hot like an acute abscess and it is therefore known as a "cold" abscess.

Amnesia—Retrograde Amnesia

Amnesia means loss of memory, and the word 'retrograde' means backwards. Retrograde amnesia occurs after a head injury (e.g. by a blow on the head by a cricketball or from a road traffic accident) and there is a loss of memory of happenings immediately before the accident.

Amputation

Removal of part or the whole of a limb is known as an amputation. Occasionally a limb is severed from the body in a severe accident. The operation of amputation may be performed (a) after severe injury when the main blood vessels and nerves have been damaged beyond repair, (b) for gangrene due to obstruction of a main artery by an embolus or by thrombosis in a diseased artery (page 9), (c) for gas gangrene caused by gas gangrene bacteria) and, (d) for a type of cancer (sarcoma) of the bones or muscles. An *'amptuation bed'* is a form of bedmaking which is used for nursing a patient with an amputation of the leg. A cradle is inserted and the bed coverings are folded back in such a way as to expose the dressings covering the stump of the leg. The nurse is therefore able to observe the stump at all times and she should report immediately any blood seen coming through the dressing. Bleeding which occurs within the first twenty-four hours of the amputation is known as Reactionary Haemorrhage because it is caused by the recovery of the patient from the anaesthetic. The blood pressure rises and this displaces the clot which blocks the end of the cut vessel. Bleeding which occurs 7-14 days later is due to infection digesting the artery in the stump and is known as Secondary Haemorrhage. The immediate treatment of haemorrhage from an amputation stump is by the application of a pressure dressing (pads of gauze and wool and crepe bandage) applied tightly to the stump. The medical staff must be informed immediately. In some hospitals a tourniquet is kept by the bed, but as its presence may upset the patient and the relatives many surgeons prefer it to be kept in one place in the ward and all nurses are instructed where to find it in an emergency.

Anaemia

Anaemia is a condition in which there is a reduction in the number or the quality of the red blood cells. In either case all the tissues of the body are affected, because red cells carry the oxygen which is needed to maintain their vital functions.

The red blood cells are formed in the red marrow of the bones, and certain substances are necessary for their formation, such as Iron and Vitamin B_{12}. The causes of anaemia are:

(1) A lack of the essential substances in the diet, or the inability to absorb them from the food during digestion.

(2) Severe loss of blood. This may be a sudden large amount as after an accident or operation, or small but repeated losses, as from piles (haemorrhoids).

(3) The person may have fragile cells which are easily broken down by the spleen. This is an inherited condition. On the other hand the cells may be quite normal, but they are broken down too quickly (haemolysed), often by the spleen. This is an acquired condition.

(4) In rare cases the bone marrow fails to produce new cells. This is either due to some poison or because of reasons unknown.

Symptoms and Signs: All or any of the following may be present: fatigue and breathlessness after any exercise or work, pale skin and mucous membrane, palpitations, indigestion and even vomiting, headache, dizziness, fainting attacks, and lack of concentration.

If the cells are being broken down too quickly, the patient's skin may have a yellow colour—jaundice. This is due to the pigment which is liberated from the cells and which is normally excreted by the liver into the bile. In this condition more pigment is liberated than can be excreted and therefore jaundice is apparent.

Laboratory Investigation: A small amount of blood is taken to be examined in the laboratory, as this helps to decide the cause of the anaemia (e.g. iron deficiency, Vitamin B_{12} deficiency). It can be seen whether the cells are abnormal in shape, colour, size and number. Examination of the bone marrow may be carried out by the doctor to find out if the cells are being produced normally. The marrow is usually taken from the sternum by means of a special needle and syringe (sternal puncture).

Treatment: (a) If anaemia is due to a deficiency of certain substances, these may be given in the diet or by injection. In some cases, where the patient is not able to absorb an essential substance, (e.g. Vitamin B_{12}) he may have to have injections for the rest of his life.

(b) If the anaemia is due to the loss of blood, this must be stopped. A blood transfusion may be given to help the patient's blood.

(c) If the cells are being broken down too quickly, the spleen may have to be removed (splenectomy) as this is the organ that destroys many of the red cells.

Nursing Points: When the patient is very ill from the anaemia the nursing is specially important. He must rest, so that the oxygen which is in the blood can be used by the vital organs instead of by the muscles. The diet must be adequate and appetising but must be easily digested since the digestive tract is not able to deal with large, heavy meals at this time.

As the anaemia affects the vitality of the tissues, special care must be taken of those areas of skin where pressure sores can occur.

Anal Fissure

A fissure is a narrow crack and in this case it occurs in the wall of the anal canal. Nearly always it follows a bout of constipation when hard dry faeces are passed. Sometimes, in the middle aged or elderly, it occurs with cancer of the anal canal.

An anal fissure is extremely painful and the pain is brought on each time the patient has his bowels open, and it may last several hours. Because of the pain the patient is afraid to pass a motion and the faeces become even harder and dryer, so causing more pain.

Thus with the treatment of these cases the prevention of constipation is very important. A substance containing cellulose (methylcellulose) is frequently given to provide a soft bulk to the faeces, or liquid paraffin (one tablespoonful on alternate nights). Too much liquid paraffin is to be avoided. In addition an analgesic ointment (ointment containing a local anaesthetic) may be ordered to be applied to the anus twice a day. Twice daily warm baths are also comforting.

As surgical treatment for the fissure, the patient may be given a local anaesthetic injection, or a general anaesthetic, and the surgeon will dilate (stretch) the anus. In severe cases the fissure may be excised (cut away) and allowed to heal naturally, care being taken to avoid constipation (as described above).

Cases of cancer in an anal fissure require a major operation (see cancer of the rectum).

Anal Fistula (Fistula in Ano)

A fistula is an abnormal passage connecting two surfaces covered with skin or a lining tissue (mucous membrane). Anal fistula usually follows an abscess which has been neglected. It opens onto the perianal skin of the buttock from the lining of the anus or rectum. There is a purulent discharge on the skin, near the anus. There may be more than one fistula. It is painful when inflamed.

Treatment: This is by operation, when the infected tract is excised and the area is allowed to heal slowly from the base of the cavity outwards.

Nursing is very important. There is a danger of added infection from the bacteria which are normally found in this area. The bowel is emptied before the operation, and aperients have usually been ordered for the two previous nights. A rectal washout is given 2 or 3 hours before the patient leaves for the operating theatre and a rectal tube is passed before the patient leaves the ward. The skin around the anus, groins, and suprapubic area should be shaved, and the skin washed with an antiseptic soap. For a few days before the operation a light non-residue diet is given, and general care of the mouth, pressure areas etc. carried out. After the operation there is often severe pain and drugs are ordered to relieve this. A normal diet is allowed on the second day. The pack or dressing which is applied in the theatre is usually removed from the wound after 24 to 36 hours, and replaced by a light pack in such a way that the *edges of the skin are kept apart.* Liquid paraffin (15 ml three times daily i.e. t.d.s.) is given, beginning in the evening following the operation, to keep the faeces soft enough to avoid straining. An olive oil enema may be ordered for the 3rd day, to be given gently. A bath after each bowel action is important.

Anaphylaxis

The use of serum to give Immunity: The serum given to patients to protect them from some particular disease is obtained from an animal, usually a horse, into which large doses of organisms or toxins (bacterial poisons) have been injected. The blood of the animal reacts by making substances (antibodies) to fight the infection. Some blood is then taken from the animal and the serum is separated, to be used in preventing or treating the disease in humans. Those most commonly used were anti-tetanus and anti-diphtheria sera (rarely used now). The serum of the horse containing the antibodies is injected into the human so that he is able to have some resistance (passive immunity) to the disease. Unfortunately, at the same time, the patient's body becomes more than usually sensitive to the horse serum, as it is a foreign substance to his tissues. Therefore, if a later dose of serum is given to that patient there may be:

(a) *Anaphylactic Shock or Anaphylaxis:* This is seen very quickly after the injection has been given. The pulse becomes quick and weak, respirations are difficult, the patient is pale and collapses, and he may die unless treated quickly. The treatment is to give an injection of Adrenaline at once. Thus it is important to find out if the patient has ever had any injections of serum previously before any serum is given, and also to enquire if he suffers from any abnormal reactions, i.e. allergy. If so, he is "desensitised" by being given *very small* doses of the serum and these are gradually increased.

(b) *Serum Sickness:* This reaction is not so serious nor so sudden as anaphylaxis. Seven to ten days after the injection of serum the patient may complain of pain in the joints and malaise (feeling "not well"). A skin rash may appear and the temperature is found to be raised. He should be kept in bed until the temperature is normal. Aspirin or some other drug for the relief of pain may be ordered to ease the joints, and a soothing lotion may be used for the skin irritation. The condition is not dangerous, but the patient is often frightened by it and needs reassurance. Drugs such as Phenergan (an antihistamine drug) may be ordered, and if the rash is very severe the doctor may order an injection of cortisone which gives swift relief.

Aneurysm

An aneurysm is a bulge in the wall of an artery due to weakness. The cause of the weakness may be (a) congenital (the patient is born with it) (b) injury, (c) infection, and (d) due to degeneration from arteriosclerosis (see p. 9). Sometimes the bulge is symmetrical ⟨⟩ and is called 'fusiform', or it may affect one side of the wall and be asymmetrical |⟩ and is called 'saccular'.

The danger of an aneurysm is that the weakened wall may give way completely and the patient will die from haemorrhage.

With modern surgery most arteries can be operated upon before this tragedy occurs, providing the condition is recognised in time. In most cases the aneurysm is either removed or it is tied off at each end. The surgeon then has to replace or bypass the affected length of artery by a graft which is a knitted or woven tube of plastic fibres (e.g. Dacron).

Apoplexy or Stroke

This diaster may be caused by one of three conditions of the cerebral (brain) arteries:

(1) Haemorrhage from one of the blood vessels—cerebral haemorrhage.

(2) Thrombosis (or the formation of a clot) in one of the blood vessels—cerebral thrombosis.

(3) Embolism, (or the obstruction) in a blood vessel due to something which is circulating in the blood, and which reaches a vessel through which it cannot pass, e.g., a bubble of fat, air, clump of bacteria, part of a clot of blood—Cerebral Embolism.

In any of these cases the patient may become unconscious and there may be paralysis. This varies from a slight weakness of one part of one limb to complete paralysis of whole areas of the body. The attack may be sudden, or it may be gradual and be followed by improvement, or it may end fatally.

Investigation: The doctor usually makes the diagnosis by his bedside examination of the patient. Sometimes he will ask the nurse to prepare for a lumbar puncture. This is performed in order to obtain some of the fluid which surrounds and protects the brain and spinal cord, the cerebrospinal fluid (C.S.F.). In some cases where haemorrhage has occurred into this fluid it will be revealed in this examination.

Treatment: (1) Paralysed limbs should be supported in a good position in order to prevent deformity. Pillows, foam rubber blocks and padded splints may be used.

(2) The care of the skin over the pressure areas is very important.

As well as carrying out the routine care of the skin, the position of the patient must be changed regularly. It is usual for two or more nurses to turn the patient every two hours, so that pressure is not allowed on any area for a long period. Whilst this is being carried out, the paralysed limb must be moved, and put into its correct position.

(3) Feeding may have to be: (a) Rectal, (b) Intragastric, that is, directly into the stomach through a tube or (c) Intravenous, whilst the patient is unconscious.

A HANDBOOK FOR NURSES

(4) Suppositories or enemas may be required in cases where the control of the bowel is lost. It may be necessary to catheterise a patient who is paralysed in order to obtain a specimen of urine to test. Catheterisation is also necessary in the cases of paralysis of the bladder because it will not empty normally and can easily become distended.

(5) Physiotherapy and occupational therapy are important for these patients.

Appendicitis

The appendix is a small piece of intestine with a closed end, attached to the beginning of the large intestine (the caecum) in the lower right hand side of the abdomen (the right iliac fossa). Appendicitis is an inflammation of the appendix and it is often associated with constipation. A small piece of hard waste matter (a faecolith) can block the opening of the appendix into the caecum so that the secretions of the lining (the mucous membrane) cannot escape. An infected pool forms in the appendix, and bacteria grow in this, causing acute inflammation. The best treatment is early removal of the appendix i.e. appendicectomy.

If not treated it may: (a) settle down or resolve itself (resolution) (b) form an abscess (c) burst, allowing the infected matter to escape into the abdomen, causing peritonitis. (The peritoneum lines the abdomen and forms a thin layer round the abdominal organs, and inflammation of this lining is called peritonitis).

Appendicectomy

In a simple case the appendix is cut off after the vessels have been tied, and the wound is then closed. The patient is allowed to sit out of bed the following day, and he quickly returns to normal. In some severe cases an abscess will occur in the wound, while in others a collection of pus forms in the pelvis between the bladder and the rectum (a pelvic abscess) or between the liver and the diaphragm (subphrenic abscess).

Appendix Abscess

If an abscess is formed around the appendix the surgeon opens it and he may allow the pus to drain out through a drainage tube until the infection clears up. This is done to prevent the spread of infection by the pus (containing the bacteria) into the abdominal cavity, which would cause peritonitis. The appendix will be removed at another operation about three months later.

Ochsner Sherren Treatment: In some cases where there is no spread of infection, the patient may be kept in hospital, under observation, so that an immediate operation can be performed if this becomes necessary. The patient is nursed sitting up in bed, with a foot board, or a pillow against the end of the bed, for the feet to push against to maintain the position. Only sips of water are allowed by mouth for 48 hours, and the mouth and teeth must be kept clean. The doctor may order fluids to be given intravenously. A fluid balance chart is recorded. The pulse is recorded, hourly at first, and the temperature two hourly. No aperients or sedatives are allowed. A flatus tube is passed, as ordered, usually every 4 or 6 hours, for 10 minutes each time. If the patient complains of spreading pain, or vomits, or there is any change in the temperature or pulse, this must be reported immediately.

Arteriosclerosis (Atherosclerosis)

Arteriosclerosis means hardening of the arteries. It is a degeneration which is both a hardening and crumbling of the artery wall which occurs with advancing age. Very occasionally it occurs in younger people. It is common in patients with diabetes and the cause is obscure, but the tempo and worries of modern life, smoking and obesity, are factors to be considered as well as animal fats in the diet.

The disease narrows the arteries and slows down the flow of blood. Thus thrombosis (clotting of blood) is very likely. Should the coronary arteries to the heart be diseased the patient will have a coronary thrombosis (p. 42). If the cerebral arteries are affected the patient may have a cerebral thrombosis causing a stroke (see apoplexy p. 7). When the leg arteries are affected the patient complains of pain in the calf muscles on walking (intermittent claudication) and in severe cases gangrene of the foot will occur. With modern surgery and in suitable cases it is now possible to by-pass the length of diseased and clotted artery in the leg by a graft (often a vein graft), or the surgeon may scrape out or rebore the artery (disobliteration).

In order to locate the exact site and extent of an obstruction of an artery the doctor will request an arteriogram. This is a special X-ray of the arteries, which are injected with a substance (Hypaque) which shows on the X-ray film.

Arthritis

(a) *Rheumatoid Arthritis.* A widespread and chronic condition, of different degrees of severity. It occurs at any age, and is more common in women than men. When it occurs in children it is known as Still's disease, but it is more prevalent at or after 40 years of age. In the very old person it is known as Senile Rheumatoid Arthritis.

The condition may be mild, causing slight disability only, or very severe, leading to crippling in a few years, but there may be remissions when the disease is not so active. The onset may be sudden, but is usually gradual. The joints are mainly affected with stiffness and pain especially in the mornings, and they may become swollen and tender, starting with the fingers first in most cases and progressing through the limbs and spine. Movement is restricted and the joints may become fixed and deformed. A few sufferers become bedridden and unable to look after themselves. The general health suffers through lack of exercise.

Treatment: There is no specific cure but it is important to relieve the symptoms, maintain the functions of the joints and improve the general health. In the acute phase, rest is important, followed by movement later. Drugs may be ordered such as Aspirin, Butazolidin, Cortisone, and ACTH, to be given as ordered. Indomethacin or Naproxen may be ordered to relieve pain. A normal diet is given, routine nursing is carried out, and bed rest is advised in many cases, where splints may be applied to some of the joints. Exercises with the help of a physiotherapist are often ordered with other treatment such as heat application or baths. In some cases, when the acute stage is over, where there are deformities an orthopaedic surgeon may be asked for advice, and operation may be undertaken e.g. Arthrodesis or Arthroplasty.

(b) *Osteo-Arthritis (or Osteoarthrosis).* This is commonly seen in people over 40 years old. It is often called "degenerative", because the cartilage on the ends of the bone in the joint is worn away. Extra growth of bone around it and muscle spasm causes limited movement which is painful. The condition may be caused by earlier damage to the joint by injury or disease and is often due to the patient being overweight. The hips and knee joints are most commonly affected, but any joints may be involved. Pain occurs on movement, especially after resting the part and in cold damp weather. When it is seen in the fingers the end joints may be swollen (Heberden's nodules).

Treatment: A reducing diet will be ordered if the patient is overweight. Local warmth and exercises will be helpful in early and mild cases. Drugs such as Aspirin, Butazolidin, the cortisone group may be ordered. A very painful joint may be supported by a splint or plaster. In severe cases the surgeon may operate to relieve the pain by:

(i) Arthrodesis—which fixes the painful joint.

(ii) Arthroplasty to reorganise or reconstruct the joint.

Arthritis may also be of specific infective origin, such as in tuberculosis, which is seen mainly in young children. Treatment is then ordered for both the infection and the joints. The specific drugs are ordered together with physiotherapy and splints to prevent or correct deformity. The affected joint may become almost fixed by fibrous (scar) tissue. This called fibrous aukylosis.

Acute Septic Arthritis occurs when organisms such as staphylococci and streptococci are carried to the joint by the blood or invade directly from a wound. The patient may be very ill with high fever and rigors. The joint, usually only one, is acutely inflamed with swelling, tenderness and pain. Pus may be present. Antibiotic drugs will be ordered, and the joint drained if necessary by aspiration or incision. The joint may become fixed by the formation of new bone. This is called bony ankylosis.

Arthrodesis. This is an operation undertaken to relieve painful joints, in severe cases, such as osteo-arthritis. The joint is completely immobilised and may be fixed by a special nail, or a bone graft, so that the part is permanently stiff.

Arthroplasty. This is surgical treatment of various kinds, to reorganise a joint where there is severe pain—most frequently the hip joint. i) Cup Arthroplasty. The end of the bone may be reconstructed and covered by a metal cup (of vitallium). ii) Replacement. The head of the femur may be partially removed and replaced by a metal artificial part i.e., a prosthesis. iii) Excision. The joint surfaces are excised and replaced by an artificial joint (a prosthesis). In the case of the hip joint the operation is known as a Charnley, a McKee Farrar or a Ring arthroplasty.

Ascites
This is an abnormal collection of fluid in the peritoneal cavity i.e. the abdominal civity which is lined with peritoneum. It is frequently part of general oedema in chronic heart disease and sometimes in kidney conditions. It also occurs in liver diseases—carcinoma or cirrhosis—as in both cases pressure is caused on the portal vein, carrying a large amount of blood to the heart. Another less common cause is tuberculous peritonitis. In cases due to heart disease, tapping of the abdomen (paracentesis abdominis) may be carried out. In this case the doctor inserts a needle through the abdominal wall into the fluid and it is allowed to drain away slowly. The legs may be similarly swollen with excess fluid, and they may be tapped, but this is not usual these days, as potent diuretics may be used.

Atheroma
Usually found in elderly patients, and is patchy degeneration in the walls of large arteries, due to arterio-sclerosis.

B

Boils

A boil is caused by infection of the root (or follicle) of a hair, and it starts as a small pimple which itches. It becomes larger, and the area around becomes hard and painful. Pus forms, and there is a yellowish discharge, which eases the pain. In a day or two the central part of dead material (known as the core or slough) comes out. After this, healing takes place quickly. A boil should not be squeezed, as this may cause the infection to spread. It is better to clean the surrounding skin with an antispetic, and no dressing is used until it starts to discharge.

Brain Abscess

An abscess may form in the brain after a deep wound of the skull, or it may follow infection in some other part of the body, e.g. the ear or the lungs.

The abscess is drained by the surgeon, who draws off the fluid with a syringe and needle. At the same time, he will inject a suitable antibiotic drug into the area, to destroy any remaining bacteria.

Burns and Scalds

Burns are caused by dry heat, such as fire or electricity. Scalds are caused by moist heat, such as hot water, fat, oil etc. The burns which result from these injuries and the treatment are similar, and so are described together.

Most deaths following burns and scalds are due to the shock, and the amount of shock is related to the amount of body surface which is involved and not to the depth of the burn, because of loss of fluid from the area. If more than $\frac{1}{2}$ of the surface of the body is burned, the shock will be very severe and may be fatal, even if the burn is only skin deep.

Burns are described as (a) superficial, when part of the thickness of the skin is destroyed (b) deep, when the whole thickness of the skin is destroyed.

Shock: Shock is the most serious complication, and is to be treated immediately, even before the injury is attended to. As in any shock, the blood in the circulation is decreased, and much fluid is lost from the body by seepage from the burnt surfaces and in the blisters. On admission intravenous fluids (usually plasma) are started immediately. They are given more quickly at first and then continued more slowly for 24 to 48 hours. The patient's blood will be grouped and cross-matched as a blood transfusion may also be given.

Because of the loss of blood from the circulation, it may be necessary to give the patient oxygen, because it is the red cells of the blood which carry the vital oxygen to the tissues.

Sepsis Prevention: Whilst the shock is being treated, the burned areas will be covered with sterile towels or sheets, because infection (sepsis) is another great danger. Because the surface of the skin is destroyed, a raw moist area is exposed and bacteria find this ideal for growth and reproduction. The patient's tissues absorb the poisonous substances that are produced and this is known as 'Toxic Absorption'. Before drugs were available to kill these bacteria this was the cause of many deaths. Nowadays the doctor orders drugs to kill the bacteria, but also it is important to keep the area covered and as clean as possible until treatment can be given. The treatment ordered depends on the surgeon in charge. It may be the "open" or "exposure" treatment when the burned area is left uncovered and is sprayed with an antibiotic powder that prevents the growth of bacteria, and at the same time forms a crust which prevents the fluid from seeping away. There are no dressings to apply or remove. This is an advantage as dressings frighten many patients, especially children.

The other method is the "closed" treatment. In this case the whole area is covered with a special net-like greasy sterile dressing (tulle gras), which does not stick to the wound. It may be left unchanged for 6 to 8 days, unless the dressing becomes moist. Antibiotic ointments are usually applied and antibiotic drugs are given, usually by injection.

In many cases *skin grafting* may be necessary as soon as the patient is fit. Usually skin is removed from some other part of the body, and it is transferred to the burned area as soon as it is in a clean and healthy condition. Preparation of the part of the body skin from which the graft is taken will be ordered before grafting.

Bronchitis—Acute

This is one of the most common complaints in this country, occurring mainly in the industrial areas, especially in the winter. It is an acute inflammation of the lining of the bronchial tubes of the lung (the bronchi). There is a cough, with sputum, and a slightly raised temperature. There may be pain in the chest, particularly on coughing. Rest in bed for a short time will help the patient, and a soothing linctus (or syrup) may be ordered. An aspirin type of drug may be given for pain. Usually the condition clears up in about one week. In some cases antibiotics (e.g. Penicillin) will be ordered for the patient. Repeated and more prolonged attacks may occur each winter until eventually chronic bronchitis develops.

Bronchitis—Chronic

In this condition, the patient has more frequent and prolonged attacks of bronchitis. Eventually he is never really free from it except perhaps for a few weeks in the summer. It causes distress and disability and may lead to serious complications, such as heart diseases or pneumonia. It is also quite common for a patient with chronic bronchitis to develop emphysema, a condition in which the walls of the air spaces (alveoli) in the lungs lose their elasticity and are not able to ventilate efficiently. Therefore, the necessary amount of oxygen is not taken in, and the carbon dioxide is not breathed out (CO_2 retention). Fog, smoky atmosphere, quick changes of temperature, smoking, all seem to make the patient worse, and they are liable to bring on an attack of coughing. These precipitating factors should be avoided as much as possible.

Treatment: There is no definite curative treatment, but smoking should be stopped or drastically cut down. A cough linctus may be ordered and tablets given for the relief of the spasm which always occurs in the muscle of the bronchial tubes (the bronchi). Antibiotics may be ordered in a severe attack.

The nurse must help the patient to live within his disability, by explaining the necessity to follow the doctor's instructions and to carry out the breathing exercises which the physiotherapist will teach him. The Medical Social Worker may also be able to help if his home conditions are difficult.

Bronchiectasis

In this condition some of the bronchial tubes (bronchi) in the lungs become dilated. This may be due to: (a) obstruction by a plug of sticky mucus, (b) something which is breathed in accidentally (a foreign body), (c) inflammation and swelling of the bronchial lining (the mucous membrane), (d) because an enlarged lymph gland is pressing on it from outside or, (e) finally, to a scar of the surrounding part of the lung. The part behind the obstruction becomes dilated, as the mucus within it collects and is stagnant and easily infected. There is a chronic cough, particularly in the mornings, and when the patient changes his position large quantities of the accumulated sputum are coughed up. This sputum is often thick, greenish in colour, and offensive to smell. In some cases there may be some blood in it. The patient is often short of breath as the lungs are not working fully. These symptoms gradually worsen.

It may be noticed that the ends of the fingers are thickened. The reason for this is not understood, but it is a condition which is seen in some chronic infections and in carcinoma of the bronchus and it is known as "clubbing".

Treatment: Postural drainage is carried out (see p. 61, section on lungs), and the nurse may be asked to assist the patient with this when the physiotherapist is not present. X-ray pictures are taken of the chest and a bronchogram is often done. This is an X-ray which is taken after a special substance has been injected which shows up the bronchi on the film.

A course of antibiotic drugs may be ordered especially for any fresh infection of the respiratory tract. In suitable cases, part of the lung may be removed by operation (lobectomy or resection of a segment).

Bronchopneumonia

The patient with bronchopneumonia has patches of inflammation in his lungs, (or in one lung only, but this is not so common.) This condition may follow bronchitis, any respiratory infection, or any acute fever. The temperature rises, as do the pulse and respiratory rates. The patient becomes gravely ill, looks blue (cyanosed), and has a cough. This kind of illness is liable to develop in an unconscious patient, or after an operation (especially on the chest or abdomen) whilst the patient is lying still in bed. It is the duty of the nurse to try to prevent this from happening. For example the position of the patient should be changed regularly. He should be well supported on pillows in a sitting position, if possible.

Inhalations may be given to help the patient cough more easily, and a sputum container should be at hand.

Treatment: The germs (bacteria) that cause the condition are present in the sputum, a specimen of which must be collected and sent to the laboratory. A sample of blood may also be asked for. An antibiotic drug will be ordered, and this may be changed to another antibiotic when the report on the sputum returns from the laboratory. Oxygen may have to be given when there is difficulty in breathing (Dyspnoea). As sleep is important, a sedative may be ordered to be given at night.

A HANDBOOK FOR NURSES

Pain in the chest can be eased by the application of a kaolin poultice. Physiotherapy is useful, and the nurse may be asked to help the patient with breathing exercises etc., under the supervision of the physiotherapist.

Bronchial Carcinoma

Cancer of the lung is really a cancer of the bronchus. It is becoming more common, especially in middle aged people and in those who are heavy smokers.

A cancer is a group of cells, growing wildly, (like weeds in an untended garden) and they invade the organs of the body, press on nerves, and push other structures out of their normal positions, and so hinder the functions of other parts. Pieces of these groups of cells may break off, and be carried in the blood stream, or lymph, and reach any other part of the body, where they settle and start new groups of cells which are called secondary growths or metastases.

The growth in the bronchus causes a cough by irritating the lining (mucous membrane). As it grows, it narrows the bronchus and prevents the mucus from being expelled, and so a pool forms behind the growth, which itself becomes infected. Small blood vessels may be broken into by the growth and any sputum which is coughed up may contain blood. There is some pain in the chest. A chest X-ray will probably be ordered, and the bronchus may be inspected by means of a bronchoscope. At the same time, if any growth is seen, a piece may be removed for examination (biopsy).

Treatment: Operation (pneumonectomy or lobectomy) is the only satisfactory treatment, and this is only successful if the condition is found in its early stages. Antibiotics may be ordered if there is any infection in the lungs. If operation is not possible, a course of radiotherapy (deep X-ray) may be given and some drugs ordered.

Buerger's Disease

This is most commonly seen in young men, when the blood vessels in the legs are inflamed, and there is some thrombosis. Cramp-like pains are complained of on walking, and the pain is relieved by resting. This is known as Intermittent Claudication and it is similar to the pain suffered by older men who have atheroma of their arteries. The pain tends to come on whilst the patient is walking, and gradually the distance that he can walk without pain becomes less. In many cases the modern operations of artery grafting cannot be performed and only *sympathectomy* (see p. 82) may be of value for a time. Smoking should be forbidden. Amputations are often required.

C

Cancer (Carcinoma)
Cancer is a malignant tumour, an abnormal overgrowth of tissue in a part of the body. It is harmful because of its ability to spread. Parts of it may get into the blood circulation and be carried to other parts of the body, forming other growths, which are called "secondaries" or "metastases". It can be likened to weeds in a garden, which grow very quickly, and if not removed smother all the plants growing there. The cancer is not enclosed in a surrounding envelope and therefore it spreads into the tissues around. It also invades the lymphatic system, therefore the lymphatic glands become included in the area which requires treating. It is thought that normal tissues may be irritated by some agent (such as certain chemicals, gases, cigarette smoke) causing them to start to grow in this abnormal and wild way. Much work is still being carried out, to find the causes and cure.

Once a malignant tumour (tumour means 'swelling') has developed in the body, it grows at a much faster rate than the normal body cells, and so pushes the tissues and organs out of its way. The pressure exerted by the tumour may squeeze blood vessels, so decreasing the circulation to the part.

Treatment: The most important point is for an early diagnosis to be made when a cancer is suspected. A nurse should always encourage the patient to report any unusual swelling or lump to the doctor, and any other signs, such as bleeding from the vagina after the periods have ended (post-menopausal bleeding), or bleeding from any other part.

On admission, a patient with any suspicion of the presence of cancer, may have part of the affected area removed to be examined under the microscope by the pathologist (a procedure known as a biopsy). The pathologist is able to tell whether the cells are malignant or not, in most cases.

The early growth, if malignant. will be removed immediately (excision) or given radiotherapy, or both. Radiotherapy may be (a) X-rays

C A HANDBOOK FOR NURSES

(b) Radium (c) Radio-active Isotopes. When radiotherapy is used, special precautions are necessary and in many cases the patient is nursed in a special department.

If the growth has passed the early stages, an operation may be carried out to keep the patient free from pain and to make life more comfortable, even if the condition is incurable. This is known as palliation.

The nurse must build up the patient's faith in her doctor and the treatment, and should the patient appear to be afraid of the future the doctor should be told. The nurse must never tell the patient that the disease in incurable, even though she may believe that it is. Calm, confident nursing is important and the patient should be encouraged in any interests such as Occupational Therapy, reading, listening to the radio etc. Visitors are allowed to come frequently.

Carbuncle

A carbuncle is formed when many hair follicles are infected, so that it looks like several boils together. The most common place for this to be seen is at the back of the neck, and it is liable to develop in diabetic patients. The central slough or core is large, and cannot escape through the small openings at its surface. The mass of dead tissue presses on the skin and hinders the blood supply so that it breaks down eventually, and later some of the skin comes away. A large open area is then left, which heals slowly, unless it is cleaned surgically by cutting away the dead tissue. Skin grafting may be necessary.

Any patient who suffers from boils or carbuncles should have the urine tested for sugar as he may be a diabetic without knowing it.

The treatment of a carbuncle is by antibiotic drugs. Sometimes the surgeon may order fomentations to be applied, or he may incise it (open it with a scalpel) or excise the dead tissue (see above).

Cerebral Compression

Compression of the brain may follow concussion. It is usually due to bleeding from an artery either within the brain, or in relation to its covering of dura mater. Thus a collection of blood under the dura mater is called a sub-dural haematoma and that between the dura and the skull an extra-dural haematoma. It is necessary for a surgeon to open the skull (burr-holes and craniotomy) to remove the haematoma and to control the haemorrhage in order to stop the increasing pressure on the brain substance.

Observations: The patient becomes drowsy and then unconscious. The pulse is full and slow but if it increases in rate the patient is in great danger. Likewise, the pupils, at first constricted, will become dilated if paralysis of the brain is being caused by the increasing size of the haematoma. Thus special charts are provided in hospitals for observations to be made and recorded every 15 minutes of the level of consciousness, the pulse rate, the pupil size and reaction to light, the blood pressure, temperature and respiration rates. If there are any movements of the limbs, or if the patient has any fits a record is made, and the facts are reported.

The airway must be kept clear at all times. Dentures will have been removed and stored safely. Suction of the mouth and nasal cavities may be required. In some cases a tube may be passed into the trachea (endotracheal) and if breathing is still unsatisfactory in long-lasting unconsciousness a tracheostomy may be performed. This is an opening into the trachea, at the front of the neck, and a tube is placed in position and secured, so that air can pass in and out. This requires careful attention. If the respiratory centre in the brain has been damaged, artificial respiration with a ventilator (e.g. Cape) may be required.

The unconscious patient is nursed flat in bed, or with one flat pillow, and is turned every 2 hours to prevent bed sores. When consciousness returns he may have another pillow. Some patients become very restless and noisy, and some form of restraint may be required to prevent them from harming themselves. The bladder should be emptied, by catheter if necessary, and bowel action may be encouraged by the insertion of suppositories, as ordered by the doctor. This may be every 2 or 3 days, if the patient remains unconscious. Fluids may be given through a Ryle's tube, or intravenously. High calorie foods can be added to maintain nutrition e.g., milk, strained beaten raw egg, and vitamins may be given. Periodic samples of venous blood are taken to test its chemical composition (electrolyte composition), as it may be disturbed. Antibiotics will be ordered in cases of wounds to the scalp, when there is discharge of cerebrospinal fluid from the nose or ear, and if there are any lung complications. A ripple bed is useful in prolonged cases of unconsciousness: it is a pad, placed under the bottom sheet, which causes frequent changing of the pressure areas, as it contains air cells. A pump is attached to the pad (usually placed at the bottom of the bed) and this controls the changes of pressure in the air cells, so changing the pressure on the patient.

Cholecystitis

Inflammation of the gallbladder is known as cholecystitis, and it is most often seen in middle-aged women who are overweight (obese) and have had many children (the "fat, fertile females of forty"). During an attack the patient feels very ill and has severe pain across the upper abdomen and under the lower edge of the right ribs. It may cause her to collapse. There is loss of appetite, vomiting, a raised temperature, and although the patient feels hot, she may have attacks of shivering (rigors.) There may be a yellow colouring of the skin (jaundice) if there is a stone in the common bile duct. The treatment is to remove the gall-bladder (cholecystectomy) in most cases.

GALL-STONES may be caused by bacteria which have infected the wall of the gall-bladder. Substances from the blood and liver (cholesterol and bile pigments) are laid around a small clump of bacteria or septic matter, so forming a stone or several stones. Gall-stones tend to block the bile ducts leading from the gall-bladder and the liver to the duodenum. In doing so they may cause biliary colic—attacks of very severe and sometimes griping pains—across the upper part of the abdomen, accompanied by retching and vomiting.

If the gall-bladder duct (cystic duct) is completely obstructed the gall-bladder becomes distended and acutely inflamed (acute cholecystitis). If the main duct leading to the duodenum (the common bile duct) is completely obstructed the patient becomes jaundiced. This is because the colouring matter in the bile (bile pigment) which normally colours the faeces, cannot pass into the intestines and is reabsorbed into the blood. The faeces become a grey, clay colour.

X-ray diagnosis of gall-stones. Some gall-stones show up on a plain X-ray but most of them do not. These are shown by a special X-ray (cholecystogram and cholangiogram).

Cholecystectomy is the removal of the gall-bladder and is the operation usually performed for gall-stones and gall-bladder disease.

Cholecystostomy is making an opening into and draining the gall-bladder, plus the removal of stones. It may be done for extremely ill patients who would not stand a cholecystectomy. The gall-bladder is drained.

Choledochotomy and T-tube drainage. Choledochotomy is making an opening into the common bile duct for the removal of stones which may be causing colic or jaundice. A special X-ray may be performed during the operation (on-table cholangiogram) to assist the detection of stones, to make sure that all stones have been removed, and that there is a clear passage for bile to flow into the duodenum. The duct may be drained by a T-tube.

Pre-operative preparation includes the administration of *Vitamin K* to help the clotting of blood as in jaundiced patients there is a risk of increased haemorrhage. *Blood transfusion* is also made ready. *Glucose* will also be given as it helps to protect the liver.

As these are operations in the upper abdomen the patient may have difficulty with breathing afterwards. *Breathing exercises* before the operation (pre-operative) are important.

Post-operative care: When the patient has recovered from the effects of the anaesthetic she will be nursed sitting up, well supported by pillows. The patient is encouraged to become as mobile as possible in and then out of bed in order to prevent thrombosis of veins in the calf muscles and therefore to reduce the risk of a pulmonary embolus.

If a T-tube has been inserted, special care is needed to make absolutely sure that the tubing is properly fixed to the patient so that the 'T' will not be accidentally pulled out of the duct. The tubing is led to a drainage bottle and the bile is collected and measured each day. The T-tube may be left in for 10-14 days and before it is removed the end may be clamped on the preceding days to ensure that the duct is open. (If it is not open, the patient will probably complain of pain and nausea, and the temperature may rise). After the tube has been removed, it is quite normal for the bile to escape into the dressing for a few days. If this irritates the skin, the dressing must be changed as often as necessary and a protective cream applied, e.g. silicone, aluminium paste etc.

The ordinary wound drains are usually shortened every day as the surgeon orders. The nurse must report any seepage of bile or blood-stained serum from the drain or from the would itself.

Chorea (see St. Vitus Dance p. 86).

Colles's Fracture

This is a very common wrist injury in elderly people, as it is due to falling on the hand, which is stretched out in an attempt to save themselves. It is common in cold weather when there is ice on the ground. The radius, on the thumb side of the arm, is broken, just above the wrist, and the lower piece is displaced forming a lump on the back of the wrist. The position of the hand is typical after this fracture, and is known as "dinner fork deformity" because it is said to resemble the curve of a table fork.

The bones are put back into their normal positions by the surgeon (i.e. the fracture is 'reduced'), and a slab of plaster is applied to the back of the hand and forearm. For this to be done the patient has to be given a light general anaesthetic, such as gas and oxygen, or a local anaesthetic is sometimes used. The fingers are left free, and the patient encouraged to move them.

Tight Plaster: Sometimes the plaster becomes too tight and causes an obstruction of the circulation to the hand. It is essential to make sure that all patients with plasters understand that they must report back to the hospital or to their doctor immediately if the fingers become blue, numb and very painful. The plaster will have to be loosened, or removed and a fresh one applied.

Colostomy

A colostomy operation is an opening of the large intestine (the colon) through the abdominal wall. Thus the faeces are passed through the opening into dressings or a plastic bag which is fixed to the skin by special sticking plaster. A colostomy is performed when there is an odstruction of the large intestine on the left side of the abdomen or rectum or anus in the pelvis. The obstruction is normally a cancerous growth or an inflammation. The colostomy may only be *temporary* as the surgeon will remove the growth or inflammation at a second operation, and then close the colostomy at a third operation in order that faeces may be passed normally through the anus once more. The colostomy may be a *permanent* opening when the surgeon has to remove the rectum and anus for cancer (abdominoperineal operation).

Making a Colostomy: The surgeon opens the wall of the abdomen, and a loop of intestine is brought out onto the abdominal wall and stitched in position, often with a plastic rod under the loop (to prevent it slipping back). An opening may be made at the time, to allow the faeces to escape into a disposable colostomy bag which is applied. Sometimes the opening may not be made for about two days. This is to enable the wound to heal, allowing less risk of infection from the faeces. When the opening is made later, no anaesthetic is necessary, as there is very little if any, feeling in the internal organs. (The nerve supply is almost all to cause movement and secretions, not sensations). The intestine may be opened on the ward, or in the theatre, with a scalpel or a cautery.

Care of a Colostomy. When the intestine has been opened, this is a colostomy. After the operation the patient is nursed in the semi-recumbent position, well supported. The dressing may have to be changed frequently for the first few days, and this may be rather unpleasant for the nurse and the patient. It is very important to understand the feelings of the patient, and not to show distaste or dislike when carrying out this work. The patient will require help and reassurance as he will have to face the future with this problem, and the nurse must help him to adjust himself to his circumstances.

As the skin around the colostomy is liable to become rather sore it may need to be protected by silicone cream or aluminium paste. A special diet may be ordered so that the faeces will not become too liquid or too solid to pass through the colostomy. Before leaving hospital, the patient is taught how to do his own dressing to protect the skin around the opening, and to regulate the diet. He will be given instructions as to when he must attend to see the doctor; and the medical social worker will be able to help him with the many problems which he may fear. In most cases the patient can control the working of the colostomy by habit so that it is emptied each morning, and he is then free to carry on with his normal work during the day without embarrassment.

Coma. See Apoplexy (p. 7), Epilepsy (p. 33), Insulin (p. 27), Diabetes (p. 27) and Uraemia (p. 97).

Concussion

This is a state when a patient is "stunned" following a severe head injury. He may be unconscious when admitted to the ward, or may be "dazed" and bewildered if conscious. There may be amnesia (p. 2) which varies in severity according to the injury, but the actual accident is never remembered. The pulse is feeble and rapid, the skin is cold and pale, and the pupils of the eyes are dilated. There is sometimes incontinence of urine and faeces. On regaining consciousness there is headache and vomiting in some cases, but many cases recover without any further symptoms. In other cases the patients pass into a state of Cerebral Compression, either directly, or after a temporary period of consciousness called the *lucid interval*.

Coronary Thrombosis. (see page 42).

Crohn's Disease or Regional Ileitis

This is inflammation and narrowing of the ileum (the second part of the small intestine) and sometimes part of the caecum. Occasionally it occurs in the colon. The origin of this condition is not known, but it is most common in young people particularly males, between the ages of 18 and 30 years. It may be mistaken for appendicitis as in the acute stage there is abdominal pain and diarrhoea. The general health suffers and there is loss of weight, lack of energy and anaemia. There are recurring attacks of pain and diarrhoea, and there may be a constant fever.

Treatment: Bed rest and low residue diet with extra vitamins and blood transfusion may be sufficient to allow the early acute case to subside. The drug Salazopyrine may be ordered. More often, it is necessary for a surgeon to operate. The affected part of the bowel is resected (cut away entirely) and the remaining healthy ends are joined together

C   A HANDBOOK FOR NURSES

(anastomosed). Alternatively an operation to by-pass the part is carried out. Nursing after the operation is similar to that after operation for Intestinal Obstruction.

Cross Infection

Cross infection occurs when one patient becomes infected from another. This is something that every nurse must try to prevent, and her own personal hygiene is important, including short clean finger nails and the frequent washing of the hands.

As the bacteria which cause infection are very small, they can be carried in the air of the ward. For this reason a patient with a specific infectious disease is isolated, i.e. nursed apart from others.

It is important to remember that infection can be spread in many ways
- (a) Directly through the air by coughing, sneezing, speaking, dust etc.
- (b) Indirectly by hands, food, dressings, instruments which may carry the bacteria, if strict hygiene is not observed.
- (c) Carriers—(see Infectious Diseases).
- (d) Insects and Aminals. Flies and mice commonly contaminate food. Milk may carry diseases such as Tuberculosis from an infected cow, unless the milk is treated. Diseased rats contaminate water, mud, etc and if this gains access to man, a severe form of infective jaundice follows. *On a Surgical ward* where patients have open wounds strict precautions are taken to prevent cross infection. Some of these steps are:
  - (i) No dressings are removed until at least half an hour after sweeping and bed making have been completed, so that particles in the air will have settled.
  - (ii) All dressings and instruments are sterilised. The nurse wears a mask and sterile rubber gloves to change the dressing. The non-touch technique is carried out.
  - (iii) Soiled dressings are placed immediately in a *covered* receiver, a bag or a bin.
  - (iv) Movement in the ward is kept to a minimum whilst dressings are in progress.

Constipation

This is the name given to the condition when the waste matter (faeces) from the alimentary tract is retained longer than is the normal habit. The passage of the stools becomes difficult or painful, as the faeces are often hard and dry. The condition of *absolute constipation* occurs when there is complete obstruction of the intestine. In this case neither faeces nor flatus (wind) is passed per rectum.

As there are different causes for constipation the treatment in each case will be according to the cause.

The Causes:
(1) Diet—shortage of water or roughage.
(2) Habits—(a) insufficient exercise of the whole body retards the muscle action of the bowel (peristalsis). (b) Laxative medicines taken unnecessarily so tire the bowel muscle that it fails to respond to the normal stimulus. (c) Not emptying bowel when the desire is felt.
(3) Abnormality or disease—these are conditions such as cancer or obstruction which require surgical treatment.

Treatment: If the diet is found to be the cause, the doctor will order this to be altered. Foods containing roughage, such as brown or wholemeal bread, fruit, and vegetables, help to increase the bulk of the faeces in the bowel and often are sufficient.

The habits of the patient will be investigated and these should be regulated if they are not satisfactory. He is encouraged to go to the toilet at the same time each day if possible, in order that a regular rhythm is established. *However, it is worth remembering that for some people it is not necessary for the bowel to be emptied every day.* It may be quite normal to evacuate the bowel every other day or even every three or four days. If this does not cause pain and discomfort and the faeces are not hard, there is no constipation. If the patient has been taking laxatives, these will be stopped for a few days in order to give the bowel a chance to recover and act normally. Regular defaecation may follow this simple step without further treatment.

If necessary, X-ray investigations will have to be carried out to find the cause of the constipation. A barium enema or a barium meal may be ordered. Enemas, or lavages may be necessary. (Lavage = Washout)

Faecal impaction: Sometimes the quantity of hard dry faeces accumulates in the rectum and becomes so impacted that the patient cannot pass it. However, the rectum is irritated by the faeces and produces a lot of slime (mucus) which is frequently discharged through the anus. If this is stained by faeces it gives the appearance of diarrhoea. This condition is known as 'spurious diarrhoea' (spurious = false). Thus, it is not diarrhoea that the patient is suffering from, but constipation.

Cystitis

This is inflammation of the urinary bladder, and it may have spread from some other part of the urinary tract such as the kidney. It may also be caused by any condition in which residue remains in the bladder, and bacteria grow in the urine which remains in it. It is possible for cystitis to follow catheterisation—a procedure which must always be carried out most carefully. Cystitis may be present if there is a growth in the bladder.

As the female urethra is shorter than the male, bacteria can enter more easily, and the condition is seen more often in women.

The Patient: The illness often starts suddenly, with a raised temperature, shivering attacks, a general feeling of illness (malaise), and pain or aching in the loin. Often it is painful to pass urine (dysuria), which, unfortunately, the patient requires to do more often than usual (frequency).

Treatment: A specimen of urine is collected and examined in the laboratory. In most cases it is possible to collect a specimen by catching some of the urine in a sterile container while it is being passed ('clean catch' or mid-stream specimen of urine). If these methods of obtaining a clean specimen are not possible, a sterile catheter will have to be passed. If organisms are found, a report will be sent to the ward giving the type of bacteria present and indicating the antibiotic drugs which will help to destroy them (the sensitivity). The doctor will order the antibiotic drugs, and often other medicines which alter the reaction of the urine (i.e. changes it from alkaline to acid or vice versa) so that the qacteria are not able to grow so easily in it. Other drugs may be ordered for the relief of pain. Extra fluids which are non-irritating (bland fluids such as barley water) are given, and at least 2—2½ litres per day should be taken. The extra fluid helps to wash out the bladder and so get rid of the infection and carries the drugs to it.

If any other part of the urinary tract is suspected of causing the infection, further tests will be carried out—cystoscopy (see section under 'Cystoscopy') intravenous pyelography (see p. 58 under kidney operations).

In the meantime the patient is to rest in bed until the inflammation has cleared.

Cystoscopy

This is the examination of the inside of the bladder, through an instrument known as a cystoscope. It is passed through the urethra, after a local or general anaesthetic has been given. It is a hollow tube, with a light and an arrangement of small lenses (a long thin telescope) which enables the surgeon to inspect the inside of the bladder.

D

Diabetes

Diabetes is a disease caused by a deficiency of insulin, the substance which is normally secreted by the pancreas. Insulin enables the body to make use of the sugars obtained from the food. Note that when we use the word 'sugar' here we do not only mean the sugar that we see on the dining table, but also that which is produced from the starchy foods which we eat (for example bread and potatoes) and which are converted to sugar by digestion. The final result of digestion is that the sugar and starches are converted to glucose. A deficiency of insulin is followed by an increase of sugar (glucose) in the blood and some of the excess glucose will be passed out in the urine (glycosuria). More urine will be excreted than usual (polyuria). In addition there are other substances which will be passed in the urine and these are known as ketones. One way of understanding diabetes is to think of lighting a fire with paper and sticks. We put in the paper to burn the wood and the wood in its turn will light the coal so the fire will burn to give heat (energy). If the paper is scarce or not available the wood will not be used up properly and the coal may only be charred. Thus, in the human body, the insulin makes the sugar burn up and this helps in its turn to burn the fat. If the insulin is not carrying out its work completely the glucose will not be used up and the fat (which is a rich store of energy) will only be partly burned, and ketones will be formed. Ketones are poisonous acid substances and if there are many circulating in the blood stream, the tissues of the body will be poisoned and the patient will suffer from severe acidosis and may become unconscious (diabetic coma). This is a serious complication.

Symptoms and Signs: The patient will complain of thirst, polyuria, lack of energy, loss of weight, and often irritation of the skin around the anus, and the opening of the urethra. People with diabetes often develop boils or carbuncles and are susceptible to diseases such as tuberculosis, arterial disease and infective gangrene.

Investigation: The urine is tested as soon as possible by 'Clinitest' methods to see if sugar or ketones are present. An estimation of the amount of sugar in the blood is carried out in the laboratory and the blood for this should be taken in the early morning. This test may be carried out frequently until the treatment is having satisfactory results. Another test called a 'glucose tolerance test' may be ordered to find out how much the level of sugar rises above normal in the blood before it is excreted in the urine.

Treatment: Diabetes is controlled by diet which is low in starchy foods and fats and also by insulin or other drugs. Complications such as boils are treated, often with antibiotics. The patient is taught about his diet and how to give his own injections if these should be necessary.

Insulin: There are different kinds and different strengths of insulin. The nurse has to be familiar with them and she should also be able to explain their importance to the patient who in most cases learns to inject his own daily dose. The main types of insulin are:

(1) *Soluble insulin:* This is the ordinary insulin and it acts quickly, but its effect only lasts for two to three hours. Soluble insulin is made up in different strengths as follows:—

Single strength .... 1 ml contains 20 Units.
Double strength .... 1 ml contains 40 Units.
Quadruple strength .... 1 ml contains 80 Units.

If a patient is ordered 20 Units, this can be given as 1 ml of single strength, ½ ml of double strength, or ¼ ml of quadruple strength.

(2) *Long-acting Insulin (Lente):* Some forms of insulin are prepared which are longer acting than the ordinary soluble insulin. The principal long acting preparations are:—

Insulin Zinc Suspensions (*a*) Lente, meaning slow, long acting,
(*b*) Semi lente lasts for about 12 hours.
(*c*) Ultra lente lasts for about 24 hours.

The doctor may order two different kinds of insulin to be given to one patient, and great attention must be paid to the type and strength that he decides should be used.

Diabetic Coma (Hyperglycaemia)

Diabetic Coma is most commonly seen in a patient who has diabetes but who for some reason has not taken the daily dose of Insulin or other drugs, or if he develops some acute infection. Very occasionally diabetic coma may be the first sign that a patient is suffering from diabetes. It may be brought on by an acute infection, or because the patient is given an anaesthetic but is unaware that he is suffering from diabetes. The coma is dangerous and requires emergency treatment.

The urine will contain a large amount of sugar, and the breath smells of acetone (a ketone which smells like nail varnish). The patient will have a dry skin and will be breathing deeply. A convenient aid to the recognition of a patient in diabetic coma is to remember that the 'D' of Diabetes stands for Dry skin and Deep breathing.

Treatment: The doctor orders an immediate injection of Insulin, which may be as much as 50 to 100 Units, and intravenous saline is given. More Insulin will be given if the patient does not respond and this treatment may be repeated regularly for twenty four hours and the Intravenous Saline will also be continued. Samples of blood will be taken frequently to estimate the level of sugar. If there is any other infection this will be treated, usually with antibiotics.

INSULIN COMA (HYPOGLYCAEMIA)

This is the opposite of a Diabetic Coma. The patient has either too much insulin in his blood, or not sufficient sugar. Thus it may occur if a diabetic patient has had a dose of insulin and does not take the correct or enough food after it, or sometimes if he does some extra work or exercise and so uses up the sugar.

For this reason he is taught always to carry some sugar or glucose sweets with him. He is warned that if he feels unsteady, hungry, weak, has a quick pulse, and is sweating, he should eat a few lumps of sugar to prevent the attack. He should, of course, report to his doctor.

If the patient is admitted unconscious, in a coma, the doctor will give him a solution containing glucose intravenously. Adrenalin is sometimes given to obtain a quick result, and the patient recovers consciousness almost immediately.

If he is seen before he is unconscious, sugar is given by mouth. An unconscious patient must never be given anything by mouth, as he is not able to swallow, and the fluid might get into the lungs and be fatal.

An easy way to remember the points of an Insulin coma are the three S's. 'S' in In*S*ulin, and 'S' for *S*weating, 'S' for *S*hallow breathing.

Diarrhoea

When the faeces are passed more frequently than normal, and are fluid instead of being formed, the patient is said to have diarrhoea. There are various causes for this:
(1) The Diet: may contain irritants such as unripe or overripe fruit, or certain vegetables which cause griping and increased peristalsis (bowel movements).

D A HANDBOOK FOR NURSES

(2) *Poisoning by infected food:* Food which has been contaminated by flies, mice, dirty hands, is a means of introducing acute and some serious infections into the body, such as paratyphoid, typhoid fever, dysentery.

(3) *Chemicals may cause food poisoning:* e.g. mushroom poisoning is due to a chemical present in certain mushrooms—(muscarine). Heavy metals such as arsenic and lead also cause poisoning.

(4) Other diseases of the bowel, such as ulcerative colitis.

(5) *Anxiety:* (such as before an examination) may cause diarrhoea.

Treatment: This, again, depends on the cause, which will have to be found. In many cases the diarrhoea will stop as soon as the irritating substance is excreted from the bowel.

If the cause is infection or disease this will be treated. In some cases the bowel may have to be washed out, and in other cases a sedative for the bowel may be ordered, to be given by mouth.

In nervous disease, the doctor may order general sedatives to calm the patient as a whole.

'SPURIOUS DIARRHOEA': Refer to p. 25—'Spurious Diarrhoea' is due to impacted faeces—a type of constipation.

Disseminated Sclerosis (Multiple Sclerosis)

This is a disease of the Nervous System in which scattered areas in both the brain and spinal cord are affected.

It is most usually seen to begin in young adults, more in women than men. The cause is not known and therefore no cure has yet been found. After the first attack the patient apparently recovers, but later, which may be a period of some years, there is another attack which is slightly more severe. This pattern is repeated, until gradually and maybe after many years the patient becomes quite disabled.

Because different parts of the nervous system are affected, different types of disturbances are seen. A patient will often see "double". There may be tingling or numbness of an arm or leg, a dragging foot, blurred and indistinct speech, or the inability to carry out fine movements of the fingers or hands. Sometimes the patient complains of a frequent and sudden desire to empty the bladder.

Treatment: The nursing of the patient is of great importance. The nurse must try to make a friendly and cheerful atmosphere and generally to give comfort. In the early stages, after an attack, the patient will be discharged and allowed to work, but he should be advised not to do work that is too tiring. During the attacks he is given rest in bed, but is allowed up as soon as possible. Exercises are given for any limb which shows any upset in its function. Routine nursing care, combined with tact, patience and a great deal of forbearance on the part of the nurse, are of the utmost importance, as the patient gradually becomes more and more disabled.

Duodenal Ulcer (see p. 93).

Dyspepsia

When the normal digestive processes are upset, the patient may complain of "indigestion", and this is known to the medical person as dyspepsia. It may be caused by worry, strain, anxiety, irregular meals, lack of sleep etc., but it may also be associated with an ulcer in the stomach or duodenum. The patient who complains of dyspepsia without any apparent cause should be encouraged to see the doctor. If any of the above causes are present, the diet should be regulated, and the patient advised to take regular meals and to rest. If regular meals are not possible owing to working hours etc., he should be told to carry biscuits or chocolate with him, and to take some at the normal meal times, and also to drink milk when this is possible.

Dysphagia

Difficulty in swallowing is known as dysphagia, and is present in many diseases of the oesophagus, and diseases of structures near theoesophagus (e.g. thyroid). It will also occur when there is paralysis or spasm of the muscles of the pharynx, such as is seen in diphtheria or poliomyelitis. It may also be complained of by a patient with a nervous disorder, when there is no actual disease or disorder of the throat, i.e. a functional neurosis when the function is upset by the nervous disorder.

Special Examination: X-rays may be used after the patient has been given barium sulphate to drink (a barium swallow). The oesophagus may be examined by means of an oesophagoscope, which is passed after the patient has been given a general anaesthetic. This is a hollow tube in which electric bulbs are used, and the surgeon can examine the inside of the oesophagus, suck out any fluid, and also take a piece of any tissue (biopsy) for examination by the pathologist to help with the diagnosis.

After the examination has been carried out the surgeon will decide on any further treatment. If there is cancer of the oesophagus, the growth may be cut out, and anastomosis may be carried out or artificial tubing inserted. In some cases of cancer a special tube may be passed through the obstruction and left in position (intubation) so that food can pass down to the stomach.

E

Embolus, Embolism

An embolus is a solid particle or a bubble of air which is carried round in the circulation of the blood. The solid particle is usually a clot of blood, but it can be a clump of bacteria or cancer cells, while droplets of fat (after a major fracture) constitute a fat embolus. If the particle reaches a vessel which is too small for it to pass through, it will be wedged there and it will block the vessel, so cutting off the circulation to the part which that vessel supplied. This is then known as an *Embolism*.

ARTERIAL EMBOLISM. The blood clot which becomes an embolus may begin in the chambers of the heart (in the left atrium or the left ventricle) as a result of heart disease. Part of the clot breaks off and is carried through the arteries to the point where it becomes wedged, perhaps in the aorta, the arteries to the leg, to the arm or to the brain. The part of the body supplied by the obstructed artery is therefore starved of blood. In the case of the leg gangrene may occur, while if an artery to the brain is obstructed a stroke or death will follow.

VENOUS THROMBOSIS AND PULMONARY EMBOLISM. Clotting of blood may occur in veins of the calf or pelvis after an operation (venous thrombosis). It is most liable to occur if the limbs are not exercised or if a pillow is put under the patient's knees to help support him. The leg muscles (usually calf) will become painful and there may be a slight rise of temperature. If the thrombosis blocks the main veins of the limb the venous blood cannot easily return to the heart and the leg becomes swollen (oedema). Anticoagulant drugs (Heparin and Dindevan) may be ordered to prevent further clotting, and a crepe bandage may be applied to give support to the leg and to reduce swelling (oedema).

If part of the clot in a vein breaks off it is carried up to the right side of the heart and passes into the lungs where it becomes wedged in the lung (pulmonary) arteries and thus causes *pulmonary embolism*.

PULMONARY EMBOLISM. If a large vessel is blocked there may be a sudden onset of pain in the chest, and the patient has difficulty in breathing (dyspnoea), and there is cyanosis (a bluish colour) of the lips, skin and under the nails. Unconsciousness may follow rapidly, and death often occurs in a few minutes.

If the smaller blood vessels are affected, there is sudden pain in the chest, dyspnoea, cough with blood-stained sputum, and the temperature rises in a few hours. Oxygen may be ordered immediately, and anticoagulant drugs given to prevent clotting. Other drugs, such as morphia may be given for the relief of pain. Warmth, applied to the chest helps to relieve the pain, e.g. a poultice of kaolin.

Empyema (see p. 61).

Epilepsy. Fits
A patient suffering from epileptic fits has a disturbance of the natural working of the brain in which it sends out messages to the various parts of the body to cause movements without the desire of the patient (uncontrolled movements). Often there is loss of control of the bladder and bowel and this usually occurs with a period of unconsciousness. The fit may be very short, or it may last for a few hours. It may be due to:—

(1) No obvious cause (known as idiopathic), and in many cases it seems to occur in some members of some families (a tendency which is inherited).
(2) A growth inside the skull, pressing on the brain.
(3) Irritation of the brain, by poisons in the blood.

The Patient: By some kind of warning the patient may be aware that he is about to have a fit. The warning may be a special smell, noises, or certain colours, and it is known as an 'Aura'. For example, a man may say that he can smell onions when there is no such smell obvious to the other people in the vicinity, and this particular aura may occur each time that a fit is imminent.

After the aura, the patient falls unconscious to the ground and may injure himself in so doing. His breathing stops for a few seconds and he becomes blue (cyanosed). After a few minutes the muscles start to move in convulsive spasms without any control. During this time the bladder may be emptied and sometimes the rectum as well. Saliva may ooze from the lips as a froth and it may be blood-stained if the tongue has been bitten.

In about $\frac{1}{2}$ to 2 minutes, the patient relaxes and goes into a coma for a short time. Then he wakens feeling exhausted and will usually fall asleep. He should be allowed to continue his sleep until he wakens naturally.

Should the coma last for several hours, the patient on wakening may not really be conscious of what he is doing—it is rather as though he was moving in his sleep. This is known as Post-epileptic Automatism and the patient may do strange, dangerous or illegal acts without being aware of them.

Nursing attention during a fit: The nurse must see that the patient is not in a position to hurt himself or others. While the jerky, convulsive movements are in progress, the nurse must not try to stop them but must prevent the biting of the tongue, by inserting a depressor.

Various drugs (e.g. Phenytoin Sodium—"Epanutin") are ordered for this condition, and these are given regularly to try to prevent the attacks.

F

Fractures

A fracture is any kind of break in a bone, whether the pieces remain in their correct positions or not. Even if the bone is only cracked this is still a fracture, as the bone is broken at the crack. There are two main types of fracture:

(*a*) *simple or closed* (*b*) *compound or open.*

A simple fracture is where there is no open wound associated with the broken bone. A compound fracture has an open wound which allows air to enter, and so is a more serious problem as there is great danger of infection. When a bone is fractured other structures may be damaged, and this is then known as a *complicated* fracture. An immediate operation may be necessary to arrest haemorrhage if a blood vessel is involved. In all cases of accident a thorough examination of the patient is made to see the extent of the damage and to make sure that the most serious injuries are treated first. Shock of some degree will be present, and must be treated, and further shock prevented.

Treatment: The treatment of a fracture aims at keeping the bones in their correct positions, or, if necessary "*reducing*" the fracture. This means that the surgeon sets the bone ends back into the normal position, so that they fit together again, and this is confirmed by X-rays. It may be necessary for the patient to have a local or general anaesthetic, so that the muscles relax to allow the bone ends to be moved together more easily.

After reduction the fragments are held in position until healing takes place, and this is known as *Fixation*. Splints or plaster of paris are commonly used and these are applied so that the joints above and below the fracture are included, to prevent movement of the part. The rest of the limb is given exercises to prevent stiffness. The injured part is protected for some time after the reduction has been done, so that the new bone may grow around and in the fractured part, and when this is completed, there is *Consolidation* of the union. X-ray pictures will show the bone to have completely healed, and it will eventually look normal again.

If it is not possible to get the broken ends of the bone into their correct positions by moving the bones—by traction or pulling—the surgeon may have to perform an *open operation*, and the ends of the bone are fixed together by means of a metal plate, wire, pin or nail, or by means of a bone graft.

Rehabilitation: When the fragments have been fixed together it is very important to ensure that the normal function of the part is maintained. The physiotherapist will give exercises, and the nurse must encourage the patient to carry these out regularly. Occupational therapy may also be given to help the patient to use the muscles which require special care.

Skin Traction: This is the name given to one method of maintaining the correct position of the bones. The skin is carefully prepared, and strips of adhesive plaster are applied and firmly bandaged in position. A wooden spreader is attached to the lower ends, and extension cord runs from this, over a pulley, with weights on the end.

Skeletal Traction: After a pin or wire has been passed through the bone, a metal stirrup is attached to the ends and weights on an extension cord pass from this, over a pulley. This maintains the position of the bones, and allows the patient some movement.

Nursing Points: When a bandage or splint is applied to a part, the nurse must frequently notice the colour of the part below and above, and feel to see that the skin is warm. After a plaster or splint has been applied, there is a danger that the blood circulation may be impeded by pressure, especially if there is swelling or ordema of the part. Any complaint by the patient of pain, or feeling cold must be reported and investigated. Pressure sores are a great danger, as the patient cannot move about the bed freely, and the skin must be attended regularly, and inspected.

The general health of the patient must be attended to, with a good mixed diet, plenty of fresh air, and care of the skin. The patient should not be rolled in the bed, when a limb is fractured, but at least two nurses should move him. If the patient is old, or if he has a "weak" chest, he should be propped up in bed, well supported, in a comfortable position. Deep breathing and exercises are encouraged. In the case of a compound fracture, antibiotic drugs may be ordered.

See also Rib Fracture (p. 84).

G

Gangrene

Gangrene is death of tissue, and it may be caused by the blood supply to a part being cut off either suddenly or gradually. A bed or pressure sore is an area of gangrene, as the blood supply is gradually cut off by the weight of the body pressing on the bed. Gangrene of the foot is most commonly due to **arterio-sclerosis** i.e. the hardening and narrowing of the arteries with age (p. 9). If the patient is very old, it is known as Senile Gangrene. Diabetic patients are liable to develop this form of gangrene. It is most commonly seen in the feet and legs, beginning at the toes. An embolus can cause gangrene.

When gangrene occurs the part changes colour. It feels cold and the pulse cannot be felt. Very often there is pain around the area, but often the patient has no feeling in the affected part, i.e. there is loss of sensation. Until the surgeon has seen the patient, and ordered treatment, the nurse should keep the limb up so that it is level with the body, and take the weight of the blankets on a cradle, and allow air to circulate round the limb. *No heat* should be applied and the part is kept *cool and dry*. It must be protected from injury and knocks.

FROST BITE also causes gangrene. In a disease known as RAYNAUD'S DISEASE (p. 87) the blood vessels contract too much when exposed to cold, even to slight degrees of cold in some cases. Also, CRUSH INJURIES may also be followed by gangrene, when the blood vessels in the injured area go into spasm.

MOIST GANGRENE is due to infection and it is prone to occur in a previously healthy limb which has suddenly become gangrenous.

GAS GANGRENE. This is a more severe form caused by gas gangrene bacteria which enter a wound, especially a deep wound. These germs cause thrombosis in the vessels of the damaged tissue, they attack the muscles, and produce a gas. There is intense pain and there is a discharge which has a very unpleasant smell. The disease used to be fatal, but now antibiotics, serum, blood transfusions and oxygen under pressure (in a pressurised bed or chamber) are used. If the condition is treated early it can be cured. Operation is necessary so that all the infected muscles and tissues can be removed.

Gastric Ulcer (see p. 93).

Gastritis

This is inflammation of the lining of the stomach and it may be an acute attack, such as: eating too rich a diet, heavy smoking, taking too much alcohol, or because of chemical or bacterial poisons in the food.

Some viruses as well as bacteria cause a gastritis (often called gastric influenza).

The patient complains of pain in the upper abdomen, loss of appetite, a feeling of sickness, vomiting, and sometimes diarrhoea. The temperature may be raised.

Treatment: At first, nothing is given to eat or drink, until the sickness is over. After this, fluids such as soda water, are given, then diluted milk. A hot water bottle, well protected held to the abdomen may help to ease the pain.

CHRONIC GASTRITIS may follow repeated attacks of acute gastritis. Unchewed food may also be responsible and people without the necessary teeth for good chewing may suffer from this.

Treatment: The teeth must be attended to, if necessary, and the patient encouraged to chew slowly and thoroughly. A light diet is given and rest after meals will help many cases. Constipation must be avoided.

Medicines may be ordered to correct any faults in the digestive function. In some cases the stomach fails to produce sufficient acid. One of the types of anaemia (pernicious anaemia) may be present.

H

Haemorrhoids

This condition is also known as piles, and is very common. The veins at the lower end of the anus become distended with blood. A dilated vein is known as a varicose vein, therefore haemorrhoids (or piles) are varicose veins in and around the anus. The anus is closed by a sphincter muscle, that is a circular muscle with a central opening. The haemorrhoids may be on either side of this muscle, so are known as (*a*) External when they are outside the muscle and are covered with skin. (*b*) Internal when they are inside the anus, and are then covered with the mucous membrane which lines the anal canal and the rectum.

The causes are often constipation and lack of exercise. The patient may complain of passing blood, which is bright red and very obvious, in the stools. Sometimes the patient will say that a small lump comes outside after passing a stool, and that it returns. In more severe cases the piles will come outside (they prolapse) and remain there until pushed back by the fingers.

Haemorrhoids may cause discomfort and pain. They may cause anaemia through the loss of blood, and so need treatment. Because many patients are very embarrassed by this condition, they do not seek treatment as soon as they should. However they should be encouraged to tell their doctor.

Treatment: If there is bleeding on passing stools, and no other symptom, injections may be given into the pile. This does not require the patient to have an anaesthetic, or to stay in bed, and is sufficient to bring about a cure in many cases. Injections may be given for this condition. During this time the patient should take care to avoid constipation. After each injection, he should rest for an hour or two, and afterwards avoid long periods of standing. If the piles prolapse, and especially if they remain down, it is usual to carry out the operation known as haemorrhoidectomy.

Preparation for Haemorrhoidectomy: A diet with very little residue is given for a few days before the operation, so that there will not be an accumulation of faeces in the bowel. An aperient is ordered for two days before the operation, and on the evening before an enema is usually given. A rectal wash-out is given on the morning of operation, and the patient is encouraged to walk about, until the time for the preparation of the skin. The skin preparation is carried out, as required by the surgeon.

Post-operatively: A tube may be inserted into the rectum whilst the patient is in the theatre, and this is usually removed in 24 hours, but not the dressing. The surgeon may order medicines for the patient, to keep the stools soft from the day of operation, and, in this case, the area around the anus is gently washed and swabbed with an antiseptic solution each time the patient has the bowels opened. This is also done when the dressing is changed. The diet will be of a low residue content. As pain is severe in most cases, drugs may be ordered (such as morphine) and they are given as required. Hot baths are found to make the patient feel easier, and these may be started soon after the operation, perhaps the 2nd or 3rd day. After the bowel has been opened, the patient may be allowed to sit in the bath, often on an air cushion for some time, as this cleans the area and stimulates healing.

On about the 8th day after haemorrhoidectomy the surgeon will perform an examination of the anus. The gloved finger is introduced to make sure that no excessive narrowing of the anus is occurring which might be permanent (a stricture). If there is, a perspex dilator will be ordered and the patient taught how to pass this into the anal canal each day. At his examination the surgeon also makes sure that there is no faecal impaction (see constipation p. 24). The patient is usually allowed home after the 8th or 10th day.

Haemothorax

This may follow fractured ribs, or a deep chest wound. It is a collection of blood in the pleural cavity, i.e. between the two layers of tissue (the pleura) which cover the lung and line the chest wall. There will be pain in the chest, worse on breathing at first, which eases as the bleeding increases, because it prevents the friction between the two layers of pleura. In many cases it is absorbed naturally. If the bleeding is very heavy some dyspnoea will be present and also the signs of internal haemorrhage. In this case aspiration may be carried out, or an operation to clear out the blood may be required. It may be necessary to give a blood transfusion to replace the amount lost.

Heart Diseases

The heart muscle may be damaged by such things as:—
- (*a*) Overwork—when the heart itself is working either at a greater speed than usual, or at a greater pressure.
- (*b*) Lack of blood supply to the heart muscle itself.
- (*c*) Poisons (or toxins) in the blood.
- (*d*) Bacteria.

HEART MUSCLE. When the muscle is affected, the pumping action is not normal and therefore any or all of the systems of the body may have difficulty, or be unable to work efficiently, because there is not an adequate blood supply.

For a time the heart muscle may be able to deal with the blood which is being returned to it in the veins. This is known as "Compensation". There are limits to this process, of course, but it will continue so long as the muscles and blood vessels remain healthy. If the patient develops any disease, or if the muscles or vessels are damaged in any way, the heart will show signs of failing to carry out its work and "Heart Failure" begins to show itself.

THE HEART VALVES. The lining of the heart (endocardium) may be permanently affected by rheumatic fever, or by another disease where bacteria actually live inside the heart on the valves (bacterial endocarditis). Also in old age the valves may become hardened by degeneration, and will not carry out their work efficiently.

HEART FAILURE. The valves of the heart normally prevent the blood from flowing backwards, and if they are diseased, they shrink and cannot do their work efficiently. In this case, some of the blood in the ventricle (lower chamber) may be pushed backwards into the auricle (upper chamber) instead of onwards into the arteries. This regurgitation causes congestion (like a traffic jam) in the auricles; the blood from the veins cannot get into them, so the veins also become congested with blood. This becomes worse as more blood arrives (just as more traffic causes worse jams) and so the congestion spreads. The main vein from the legs and trunk, (Inferior Vena Cava) carrying blood from the digestive tract, liver and all the other abdominal and pelvic organs become congested, and thus the liver and abdominal organs become swollen. The Superior Vena Cava, returning the blood from the head and neck also becomes congested, and the veins which run into this large vein can often be seen standing out in the neck (distended external jugular veins). The pulmonary veins, carrying the blood from the lungs become too full, and eventually this affects the lungs, and so the patient suffers from breathlessness.

When this condition is reached, it is known as Congestive Heart Failure, or Congestive Cardiac Failure (C.C.F.).

Symptoms of heart failure. In cases of heart disease the following symptoms may be complained of:

(*a*) Breathlessness on exertion at first, but later there is some degree of breathlessness even when the patient is at rest. It may be so severe that the patient is unable to breathe easily when lying down, and she has to sit up or be propped up even for sleep. Difficulty in breathing is known as dyspnoea, and in the later stage when she has to be propped up it is known as orthopnoea.

(*b*) Because of the congestion there may be: (1) a cough, and some blood may be coughed up (*haemoptysis*): (2) a blue colour of the skin, particularly of the lips and ears, due to lack of oxygen (*cyanosis*): (3) the back pressure in the veins allows some of the fluid part of the blood to escape into the tissues and so swelling occurs in the lowest parts of the body. This is oedema (often called dropsy), and if the swollen part is pressed with the finger, a dent will remain for a short time after.

(*c*) Palpitation. There is a period of rapid beating of the heart, and the patient may feel it.

(*d*) Feeling of sickness (nausea) and perhaps actual vomiting.

(*e*) Inability to sleep well, and a feeling of being irritable.

(*f*) A decreased amount urine is excreted.

Treatment: Rest is necessary for the heart, and also for the whole body and the mind. An anxious patient will not rest. All routine nursing is carried out without disturbing the patient more than necessary. *A light diet*, with limited fluids, will probably be ordered, and it may be necessary to restrict the amount of salt that the patient takes. Salt tends to retain the fluids in the body, so increasing the oedema. Because of this a *fluid intake and output chart* is kept so that all fluids that the patient takes to drink, or given by any other method, are recorded. Likewise, any fluid which is excreted must be carefully measured and recorded in the same chart, so that the doctor can see whether the patient is accumulating fluid.

Drugs: If the drug digitalis or 'Digoxin' is being given, the fluid balance chart is even more important, because the amount of urine is usually increased as the drug starts to work. For the same reason, a careful watch must be kept on the pulse rate, which is recorded regularly, and accurately. The treatment of oedema may be summarised by the three D's: Diet, Drugs, Drainage. The diet and the drugs (diuretics) are ordered as above. Drainage of fluid may be from the abdomen, chest or legs and is known as Paracentesis of the Abdomen or Chest, and Acupuncture of the legs.

HIGH BLOOD PRESSURE (also known as Hypertension or Hyperpiesis) The blood in the blood vessels is under a certain amount of pressure and this is normal.

Exercise, emotions and excitement can cause a rise in blood pressure in a perfectly healthy person, but it also occurs in some diseases, and then it can become very serious. Many people have a raised blood pressure and do not know about it. There may be no obvious signs of it until the patient is examined for some other reason.

Some people with a high blood pressure complain of throbbing headaches, dizziness, or a faint feeling on moving quickly.

The condition is most usually seen in elderly people, a normal result of growing older. As age advances, the blood vessels become less elastic or narrower and this increases the pressure.

High blood pressure can cause a strain on the heart, but one of the more common results is the bursting of a blood vessel, often in the brain (Cerebral Haemorrhage see Apoplexy). The kidneys are also damaged.

In most cases which need treatment certain drugs are given to reduce the pressure. At the same time, a sedative may be ordered to keep the patient calm and prevent an increase in pressure from excitement. As some of these drugs have other effects, the patient must be carefully watched, and a note made and reported if he complains of them. For example, the vision may be blurred, there may be constipation, dizziness, faintness or depression. These symptoms (side affects) may only last for a short time after the dose has been given.

If the cause of the high blood pressure is disease of some organ such as the kidney this will be treated, and in some cases an operation (e.g. nephrectomy) is necessary.

CORONARY THROMBOSIS

The two coronary arteries supply blood (containing the vital oxygen) to the heart muscle. If these arteries become diseased by atheroma (p. 11) a clot may form and so the blood supply to part of the muscle will be cut off. If one of the main arteries is obstructed death is sudden. If the clot occurs in a small branch of the artery only a part of the heart muscle dies.

The patient gets a sudden severe pain in the chest or arm which can last for maybe hours or days. Then the pain ceases and he begins to recover, whilst the dead tissue in the heart changes, and becomes a scar, just as a cut or operation leaves a scar. During this time there must be no strain on the heart, and the patient must be nursed at complete rest, usually for three or more weeks, in bed, until this healing is complete.

Drugs (anticoagulants) may be ordered to try to prevent any further clotting, but rest is the most important factor. Also during the first days, the doctor may order drugs (e.g. Morphine, Pentazocine) to relieve the pain, and to stop the patient from worrying.

Hernia or Rupture

A hernia is said to be present when an organ or any part of it protrudes through the wall of the cavity in which it normally lies. The types most commonly seen in hospital are of the abdominal organs, but there are other types, e.g. cerebral hernia, when part of the brain protrudes through an opening in the skull.

Abdominal herniae may be either (a) External, when the protrusion occurs through some part of the abdominal wall causing a swelling, which can be seen or felt. (b) Internal, when the protrusion of some part of an abdominal organ occurs into some other part, and can only be seen on the operating table when the abdomen is opened.

An external hernia may be present at birth (congenital), because of some weakness of the abdominal wall into which a sac of peritoneum protrudes at birth. A part of the intestine is liable to slip into the sac when the pressure in the abdomen is raised, as may occur in coughing, crying, and on straining to empty the bowel etc.

TYPES OF ABDOMINAL HERNIAE

External herniae are described according to their positions; the most common being:

(a) *Inguinal*, when the swelling is in the groin, as the protrusion is into the inguinal canal, which runs along the groin. It is more common in men than in women, because before birth the testes pass along this route from the abdominal cavity to the scrotum. The canal is wider in the male because of this, and therefore more prone to allow a hernia to develop.

(b) *Femoral hernia*. In this case, the swelling is not so near the midline of the body as in the inguinal hernia, and it is lower in the groin. The organ protrudes into the femoral canal, near the femoral artery and vein. It is more common in the female, because the canal is wider due to the different shape of the pelvis.

(c) *Umbilical hernia*. This is seen at the umbilicus on the front of the abdominal wall. It is mainly seen in babies and young children, or in fat, elderly women who have had a number of children with consequent weakness of the muscles of the abdominal wall.

(*d*) *Ventral or Incisional Hernia.* This type of hernia occurs anywhere on the abdominal wall, and is usually post-operative. It may be due to the muscles of the wall not uniting strongly, or to stretching of the scar, and is especially liable to occur after a drainage tube has been used, or if the wound has become infected.

(*e*) *Other types of herniae* are not so common, but another two which are occasionally seen are (1) Hiatus hernia, when the top part of the stomach pushes upwards through the opening in the diaphragm, normally occupied by the oesophagus. (2) Diaphragmatic hernia, when abdominal organs protrude into the chest through a hole in the diaphragm.

In many cases of hernia, the contents of the hernial sac can be pushed back, into the abdominal cavity by hand, and this is known as a *reducible hernia*.

COMPLICATIONS. If the contents of the sac cannot be returned it is said to be *irreducible*. This may be due to the swelling of the contents of the sac, or to tissues forming adhesions.

Another complication of a hernia which is very important is *strangulation*. A strangulated hernia is one where the loop of intestine is being strangled, that is, its blood supply is cut off, and the blood return by the veins is also obstructed. This leads to death of the part (gangrene). It may be caused by a ring of tough fibrous tissue round the neck of the sac which has stretched on exertion (e.g. a violent cough) to allow the part of the intestine to enter the sac, and it then contracts to its normal size, and so traps the piece of intestine. This is an emergency and an operation is necessary to save the patient's life.

The tissue which is inside the sac will die and become gangrenous if the blood flow is obstructed, and the dead tissue will be a breeding ground for bacteria, so leading to a general infection of the abdominal cavity and its lining (the peritoneum). An infection of the peritoneum is known as *peritonitis*.

In addition to strangulation of the blood vessels, the intestine is obstructed and the contents will not be able to pass along. This is one variety of intestinal obstruction.

TREATMENT OF HERNIA. In an infant, an umbilical hernia will usually respond to treatment by pad and strapping to keep the hernia under control until natural closure of the part takes place.

In an older patient, an operation is the only means of curing the hernia, but, if the patient is very old or unsuitable for operation, the hernia may be supported by means of a truss. This holds the part in position, preventing discomfort, but it does not cure.

If the hernia is reducible, a *truss* may be used to keep the hernia reduced, but an operation is necessary to cure any type (except in an infant). The *operation* may be known as (a) Herniotomy, when the hernial sac is removed (b) Hernioplasty, when a repair is carried out, by applying some tissue from another part of the patient (fascia or skin), or an artificial tissue (e.g. nylon net) to repair the region.

After Operation. The patient is usually nursed in the most comfortable position, often in the semi-sitting position. Leg exercises are an important part of the post-operative care, as well as breathing exercises. The passing of urine, and bowel action are important for the nurse to watch for and report on. If urine is not passed it may be necessary for the surgeon to order a drug to encourage this or the patient may be catheterized. In some cases, the patient is kept in bed for only 2 or 3 days, but it may be necessary for there to be 2 or 3 weeks' rest in bed. This is to allow the wound to heal properly, and depends on the operation which has been carried out. The patient is advised not to do any heavy lifting, or strain the abdominal muscles for 3 months after the operation, in order that the repair may be given the time to heal thoroughly.

STRANGULATED HERNIA. The patient will complain of pain in the area, which is severe colic which comes and goes (intermittent). There is vomiting. This starts at the beginning of the attack, recurring only at intervals. It becomes more frequent and finally is persistent. At first the stomach contents are vomited, then a greenish fluid (as in a bilious attack). Later the vomited material is brown and foul-smelling, known as faecal vomiting. There is complete constipation (no flatus and no faeces), and as the intestine is completely obstructed the abdomen becomes distended.

The patient is admitted to hospital as soon as possible as an emergency. The nurse is asked to pass a tube into the stomach, and withdraw the contents. The doctor will probably give intravenous fluids to replace the fluid lost by vomiting. The patient is taken to the theatre and an operation performed to release the strangulation. If the loop of intestine is gangrenous, it will have to be cut out (resected) and the two healthy ends joined together (anastomosis). After the return from the theatre, the stomach contents will be withdrawn through the nasogastric tube and intravenous fluids are given. When the patient is able to take sufficient fluids by mouth, and the normal bowel movements have returned, diet may be gradually introduced.

H A HANDBOOK FOR NURSES

Hodgkin's Disease (or Lymphadenoma)

The cause of this disease is not known. It affects the lymph nodes, and is most commonly seen in people of 20 to 40 years old, but may occur at any age. Any one or many groups of nodes may be affected and the first sign of the disease is often an enlargement of one group. The nodes in the neck, axilla, or groin are usually involved but occasionally those inside the abdomen or chest may be affected first, making early diagnosis difficult. The spleen and liver may be affected. There is not much alteration in the general health to be noticed at first, but gradually the patient feels weak, loses weight and becomes anaemic, and this general decline is progressive. Temperature variations may occur (Pel Ebstein's fever) rising to 40°C for 7 to 10 days and then returning to normal again for 2 or 3 weeks.

If the thoracic lymph nodes are enlarged they may cause hoarseness, cough and dyspnoea by pressure. The diagnosis is confirmed by taking out an affected lymph node for examination under the microscope (Biopsy). The surgeon may perform a laparotomy to examine the liver and spleen and the areas where lymph nodes are likely to be affected. He may remove the spleen.

Treatment: As the cause is unknown curative treatment is difficult. Nevertheless some good results are being achieved. In the so-called 'Stage One', when one group of nodes only is affected, it may be cured by radiotherapy. In widespread cases some drugs (e.g. cytotoxic drugs) may be ordered to try to cause the disease to subside.

Hydrocele

This is a collection of clear fluid in the sac (tunica vaginalis) which surrounds the testicle. A congenital hydrocele may occur if the sac is not completely closed. Its cause in an adult is not known, but it may follow disease of the testicle.

Treatment: i) Tapping. The skin is cleaned with an antiseptic solution e.g. Savlon. A torch is used to light up the swelling from the far side (transillumination) so that the surgeon can see through and avoid puncturing any of the blood vessels when he inserts a trocar and cannula (under a local anaesthetic). The fluid is allowed to drain away, and the puncture is then sealed with some collodion on gauze. This procedure may have to be repeated several times. ii) Aspiration. In this case a syringe and needle is used. iii) Operation, to prevent recurrence, may be performed.

Hysteria

In hysteria the emotions seem to control the will power, instead of the reverse. The patient then becomes under the control of her emotions, leading her to do things which she would not normally think of doing. It is most commonly seen in young women, but may be seen in boys and men. It is often made worse by disturbances which may be physical, such as at puberty or by an accident.

The patient may appear to have developed almost any form of disease, from digestive upsets, paralysis, a rash, loss of feeling in one or more parts of the body, being unable to swallow, deafness, blindness, or fits. Often there appears to be an odd kind of indifference to the symptoms (belle indifference).

Treatment: The nurse must realise that this is a real disorder and it is one which is most difficult to treat.

Sympathy for the patient should not be shown, as this is one of the reasons for the attack—an unconscious desire for sympathy. It is important also not to allow the patient to think that the medical and nursing staff know that there is no physical illness, or she will have no confidence in her nurse. It is right to treat her kindly but firmly, and to encourage her when she behaves more normally, assuring her that she will soon recover. She may make the best progress if given rest in bed, away from other patients, with fresh air and a good diet. Over-sympathising friends and relatives should be asked to leave her alone for the time being.

Hysterical Fits. If the patient has a hysterical fit, it can be distinguished from an epileptic fit by the fact that she does not become unconscious, does not pass urine or faeces, and that the fit may last for 15 to 20 minutes whilst the epileptic fit only lasts for 3 to 4 minutes.

The treatment is to loosen the clothing around the neck, open the window, and sponge the face with cold water.

I

Incontinence

Incontinence means the inability to control the natural evacuations of the body.

(a) *Urinary Incontinence.* This is often present in a very ill patient, especially if elderly. It may occur in some diseases of the Central Nervous System, and in most cases of coma. In "stress" incontinence, a small amount of urine is passed involuntarily during exertion or pressure such as coughing, laughing etc. Incontinence in an ill patient makes frequent changing of the bed-clothes necessary, and special care must be taken of the pressure areas.

There may be apparent incontinence when the bladder is full i.e., there is retention of urine with overflow, as the kidneys continue to produce urine and pass it on to the full bladder. A careful watch must be kept for this state of affairs as catheterisation will be needed, carried out with full aseptic technique. A catheter may be inserted and left in position for some time, draining into a bag or bottle. The bag or bottle can be emptied when necessary. If and when normal bladder function returns, the catheter is removed (see under Paralysis, p. 71, for catheterisation).

(b) *Faecal Incontinence.* Incontinence of faeces may be present in any very ill patient and very often in cases of unconsciousness and coma, and in mentally ill patients. It also occurs in some very old people, due to loss of muscle tone. Quite often it is a manifestation of *impaction of faeces* in the rectum, when liquid faeces constantly discharge through the anus from around the large mass of faeces above. This is called pseudo-diarrhoea (or spurious diarrhoea).

Treatment: This depends on the cause, and will be ordered by the physician. It is extremely important for the nurse to see that the patient is kept clean and in a dry bed, and to care for the pressure areas. Various drugs or suppositories may be ordered, also oil enemas and manual disimpaction in the case of impacted faeces.

Infectious Diseases or Specific Fevers

1. CHICKENPOX
2. DIPHTHERIA
3. GERMAN MEASLES
4. MEASLES
5. MUMPS
6. POLIOMYELITIS
7. SHINGLES

This term is usually used to mean the diseases which can be spread by direct contact, from person to person, and so cause epidemics. Many other diseases can be spread in this way but do not usually cause epidemics, e.g. Infective Hepatitis, Syphilis.

A HANDBOOK FOR NURSES

Various terms are used, when discussing these infectious diseases, e.g.:

Carriers—This term refers to people who carry a disease and transmit it to other people, but do not themselves suffer from the disease, that is, they are *Immune*.

Immunity—When the body is able to resist an infection, although in contact with it, that person is said to have immunity. This often happens after an attack of the disease. For example, a person may have measles as a child, and is then probably immune for the rest of his life. Immunity occurs because certain substances are built up by the body to overcome that particular germ, and these substances continue to remain in the blood always, and are ready to fight that germ if it should try to invade the body on any later occasion.

Vaccination: This is a method of giving immunity to a person. A small dose of the germs, either killed or very much weakened, or the toxins produced by them which are altered by chemicals, will cause the body to react as though it was an attack of the live germs, and so immunity results without the person being ill. For example, people are vaccinated against smallpox, tuberculosis, etc.

A short period of immunity may be given to a person by taking some blood from a patient who has suffered from a certain disease, and which contains the necessary protective substances, and giving him some of the fluid (serum) of this blood. This may be done for a very delicate child, during an epidemic to prevent him from suffering from an attack of some infection which he is not strong enough to fight. It is done, in some cases, for a woman who is under three months' pregnant and has, say, German measles, which might cause defects in the baby. This type of immunity is passive and does not last for long, but it helps the person over the period when she may be in contact with a patient, and is in danger of becoming infected, without time for her body to prepare to overcome it.

Incubation Period: When a germ enters the body, it grows and multiplies until there are enough germs to affect the patient and cause the illness. This is the incubation period, the time that elapses between the germ entering the body and the first sign or symptom showing.

There are different Incubation periods for the different infections, but each one remains more or less the same in each disease:

A HANDBOOK FOR NURSES

Incubation periods for the common infectious fevers

Short Period	Scarlet Fever Diphtheria	3–5 days
Medium Period	Typhoid Fever Whooping Cough Small Pox Measles	10–14 days
Long Period	Chicken Pox German Measles Mumps	14–21 days

Stage of Invasion: When the germ (or the poisons that it produces) have become wide-spread throughout the body, so that there are signs and symptoms of the disease, it is known as the stage of invasion.

Some of the signs and symptoms are seen in all Infectious Fevers, such as raised temperature, feeling of illness (known as malaise), loss of appetite, hot skin, dry tongue, and less urine being passed. There are other things in each fever, such as a rash, which enables the doctor to diagnose the case.

Nursing of Infectious Diseases

Any patient who is suffering from one of these diseases must be nursed away from other patients. Even before it is definitely known to be an infectious case, but is suspected, the patient will be *Barrier Nursed*.

The nurse must also take precautions to protect herself, by very carefully carrying out all the rules for personal hygiene that she has been taught. This is important, not only for her own benefit, but so that she will not become a carrier and carry infection from one patient to another. Washing the hands, after attending to the patient, when leaving the ward, and of course, before meals, is more important than ever. The hands should be kept in good condition, by drying carefully and applying a hand cream. Any sore throat, septic cut, or rash should be reported immediately.

1. CHICKENPOX (VARICELLA)

Chickenpox is caused by a very small germ (a virus) and is very contagious. It is usually passed directly from one patient to another, but may be carried on clothes. Children under 12 years of age are most likely to be seen suffering from Chickenpox. It takes 2 to 3 weeks to develop after the child has been exposed to the infection, i.e. the incubation period varies between 12 and 21 days. It may follow contact with a patient suffering from Shingles (Herpes Zoster. see p. 55).

Symptoms: The patient may not feel ill at all, and the first sign of the disease is the rash on the trunk, and maybe on the scalp. The face and limbs are never so much involved as the trunk. There may be only a few spots, or quite a lot. They begin as small pink round or oval raised areas of skin (vesicles) with fluid beneath. These soon wither away and become scabs or crusts. All the stages of the rash can be seen at the same time, as they appear in crops.

Treatment: No special treatment is necessary. Scratching must be prevented, and the rash kept clean. The child may be kept in bed for a few days, and the itching relieved by sponging with a mild antiseptic (boric lotion). If the rash becomes infected, drugs may be ordered to fight this secondary infection. There are no drugs which are effective against these virus infections.

2. DIPHTHERIA

Diphtheria is not seen often now, thanks to the inoculation of children, which every nurse should encourage. The disease is caused by a germ which enters the body and remains in one place, but the powerful toxins (poisons) which it makes travel round the body causing serious effects.

The most common sites for the bacteria to settle are the throat (Fauces) and the nose. Sometimes the larynx, at the top of the trachea (wind pipe) may be affected, either directly, or by spreading from the nose or throat. Where the germs settle, an exudate or membrane is formed which looks yellowish in colour. If this is the larynx it may obstruct breathing, in which case an emergency operation may be necessary known as a *Tracheostomy.*

Symptoms: The patient feels tired, cold and "shivery", but there is *no* complaint of a sore throat, in many cases. The temperature may be slightly raised for the first 1 or 2 days but then returns to normal, even if the infection is spreading. In nasal diphtheria there will be a discharge from the nose which may be blood stained.

Treatment: The doctor will give diphtheria antitoxin even before the disease is definitely diagnosed. A throat or nasal swab will be sent to the laboratory for testing. Whilst awaiting the results of these tests, treatment will be given for diphtheria, because this may save the life of the patient, and will not harm him, even if the results of the tests show that the cause of the illness is not diphtheria.

Nursing is important as the toxins may cause heart failure. The patient should be isolated and nursed in a warm room, lying almost flat for 2 to 3 weeks. He should not be allowed to exert himself, and should be moved gently. The diet will be of nourishing fluids with glucose only, at first, and a light diet will be introduced gradually. Treatment of the mouth and pressure areas must be carried out regularly. Small daily doses of liquid paraffin may be ordered to prevent constipation, and a small enema given every 3 or 4 days if necessary, in the early stages of the disease.

If in addition a tracheostomy is performed for laryngeal obstruction the nurse will have the additional responsibility of the care of the patient with this artificial opening into the trachea. She should familiarise herself with all the details of management as taught her in the classroom and by reading the appropriate textbooks.

Complications which may occur are serious, and the nurse must watch for signs of them.

(1) The heart may be involved. As this will cause an increase in the pulse rate an *accurate* pulse chart must be maintained. The patient will look pale and grey, and the output of urine will be decreased.

(2) *Nerve damage:* Paralysis may develop in almost any of the muscles. The ones most commonly involved are those of the throat (pharyngeal muscles). Speaking and swallowing are affected, and fluids may come down the nose, when drinks are taken. It is important to watch for any signs of these complications and report them immediately. Occasionally the muscles used for breathing (intercostals and diaphragm) are affected, causing such difficulty in breathing that an 'iron lung' (mechanical respirator) will be required. If the eye muscles become paralysed the patient will complain that he is unable to see clearly for reading etc. There may also be areas of skin in which the sensation is lost. This paralysis, (both movement and sensation) is temporary, the functions and feelings return gradually to normal on recovery from the diphtheria.

3. GERMAN MEASLES

This is less infectious than Measles, but, as it may affect an unborn baby if the mother has the disease in the first few months of pregnancy, girls are often allowed to come in contact with a case so that they become infected before they are married, and so, after having an attack of the disease, they develop an immunity.

There is a long incubation period, and the rash is often the only thing that lets the patient or her family know that there is any illness. The spots are small and pink, becoming raised, but they do not run into each other as in Measles. There are no Koplik's spots. The rash disappears in about three days. Lymph glands at the back of the ear may be swollen.

No treatment is necessary.

4. MEASLES

This is more common in children than adults, and is most often seen between the autumn and spring, i.e., October and May. It is caused by a virus, which is smaller than a bacterium, and may be spread by direct contact with a patient, by coughing and sneezing, that is, by droplet infection.

It takes between 7 and 21 days for the viruses to grow in the body. After this incubation period the child appears to develop an ordinary cold, with a raised temperature, running nose and eyes, sneezing and coughing. During an epidemic of measles, the nurse should look inside the child's mouth, as, during this stage, there will be small greyish spots on the inside of the cheeks near the back teeth, (if it is a case of measles). These spots are known as Koplik's spots, and are a sure sign that it is not a common cold, but a case of measles. On the third day, the child will appear to be better, and the temperature is normal again, but the next day, the rash will appear. This starts as flat, pink spots, behind the ears, and then spreads quickly, over the face, body, arms and legs. The spots run into one another, and become a darker colour, and the temperature rises again. After a few days the spots fade, the temperature returns to normal, and peeling of the skin often follows.

Treatment: The patient is isolated from others, and kept in bed until the temperature has returned to normal, in a shady, or darkened room, which is well ventilated. The nose and mouth must be kept clean, and a note made, and reported should there be any discharge from the ears, as they may be involved in the infection.

The child may have to be propped up in bed, if there is a cough, in order to avoid Broncho-pneumonia, which is a complication of measles, particularly in very young children. Nowadays, inoculation is given to prevent this.

A HANDBOOK FOR NURSES

Sponging may be carried out with warm water if there is much sweating, and the clothes are changed as often as necessary. The clothes should be light in weight and not irritating to the skin.

If there is no appetite, plenty of fluids should be given, but, as soon as the temperature is normal, the usual diet can be taken. The doctor may order drugs for the patient. These are not to treat the measles, but to prevent such things as broncho-pneumonia.

The patient will be allowed to get up, probably by the end of the first week. He has to stay in his room, and the doctor will allow him to be with other children after two weeks, unless there are signs of any complications. After recovery, the child needs a time to recuperate, and a holiday should be arranged, if possible, or a short time at a convalescent home.

5. MUMPS (EPIDEMIC PAROTITIS)

Mumps is caused by a virus, and is most common in children between 6 and 16 years of age, particularly boys.

The incubation varies between 1 and 4 weeks, most often about 18 days.

Symptoms: The child feels ill for one or two days, before a swelling is seen. This appears below the ear, in the parotid gland (which helps to form saliva). One side usually swells first and is tender to touch. The other side follows in 2 to 4 days. The glands under the jaw (submaxillary) often swell too. The temperature is raised to 100° to 101° F. Swallowing may be difficult, and even opening the mouth may be painful. The swelling usually begins to go down after a week or ten days. In boys, usually after puberty, the testicles or ovaries may become inflamed and painful (orchitis), causing permanent damage in a few cases.

Treatment: The patient is kept in bed for at least 10 days. Semi-solid foods, such as custard, are easier to swallow than fluids, for which a straw may be helpful. Aspirin may be ordered to relieve pain, and help in keeping the mouth clean. Poultices may be applied to the glands. If the testicles are swollen a wrapping of cotton wool is applied, and support may be given by a small sandbag or rolled-up towel.

6. POLIOMYELITIS (INFANTILE PARALYSIS)

This is an infection of the nervous system by a virus, which affects the nerves controlling the movement of various parts of the body. It is thought that many people have mild attacks and are not ill, but develop immunity to the disease. Other people have the infection, but do not have any serious signs or symptoms, and other patients are ill but do not have any paralysis. It occurs in epidemics, usually at the end of the summer, and the method of spread is not certain, but the virus is in the faeces of the patient, and is also found in the throat, and can therefore be spread by droplets. If the faeces are exposed, flies may carry the infection to food, also. Because of these factors, it is important for the nurse to realise the importance of washing her hands after touching anything belonging to the patient, after attending to him, and, also, seeing tha tothers carry out the same precautions. A separate bedpan should be kept for the patient.

Immunisation: It is important to encourage people to have immunisation against poliomyelitis. The vaccine can now be given by mouth, instead of by injection which many people avoided. It is routine to give 3 doses, at monthly intervals, and another dose (booster) later. In this way, the disease can be prevented from becoming epidemic.

7. SHINGLES (HERPES ZOSTER)

Shingles occurs following a virus infection of the root of a Spinal Nerve (i.e. a nerve given off from the spinal cord in the backbone). Vesicles appear as in Chickenpox, but only on the skin which covers the path of the infected nerve, usually in the chest and abdominal regions. It may be on the face when one of the upper nerves is affected, and this may have more serious results. The disease is very painful, and sedatives are often ordered. Dressings may be applied to soothe the pain in the area. Herpid, a special preparation, may be applied. Shingles is more distressing when it occurs in an elderly patient, because of post herpetic neuralgia.

Infective Hepatitis

This is inflammation of the liver caused by a virus, and the condition sometimes occurs in epidemics, being passed from one person to another, either by the faeces or by flies. The virus is present in the patient's blood and it can be passed to others via non-disposable syringes used for taking samples of blood. Disposable syringes should be used, as chemicals do not destroy the virus. If non-disposable syringes are used they should be sterilised by dry heat in an autoclave, just as dressings are.

The Patient: He feels ill and there is a slight rise in temperature. He feels sick and may actually vomit, or there is a loss of appetite, especially for fatty-foods. Abdominal pain may be present. After a few days the patient often feels better and it may be then that the jaundice appears.

A HANDBOOK FOR NURSES

The patient may complain of itching of the skin, but this is not so intense as that itching which occurs when the bile ducts are obstructed by gall-stones or by a cancer of the pancreas.

Treatment: Rest in bed is important. The patient tires very easily and for some weeks afterwards may feel exhausted.

Diet: Glucose and fruit drinks are given and, as soon as the patient will take food, proteins should be introduced (e.g. eggs, fish, chicken, meat) to help the liver to overcome the infection. The doctor may order extra vitamins, and the diet will continue to have only a small amount of fat in it until he is completely recovered. No alcohol is allowed for 6 months.

Isolation: All steps must be taken to prevent the spread of infection. The nurse must attend to her own hygiene, especially washing her hands after carrying out any nursing care for the patient. All food must be protected from flies, but this is important at all times. Soiled linen is treated as infected, and, when handling bed pans, the nurse should wear rubber gloves which are sterilised each time after use.

Patients who have had this disease will not be allowed to give blood as blood donors, and they should always be told of this.

Insulin (see p. 27).

Intestinal Obstruction

This term is applied to a complete stoppage of the passage of the contents of the intestine. It is particularly serious and a danger to life, if not treated immediately. The fact that some patients do not appear to be very ill at first is an added risk. The temperature remains normal, and the pulse may be normal, or only slightly raised.

Symptoms and Signs: There is some *abdominal pain* in the central part of the abdomen, and this comes and goes in waves, until the obstruction is relieved or the intestine becomes paralysed. *Vomiting* always occurs. At first, the food from the stomach is returned, then a greenish bile-stained fluid, and later, the contents of the lower part of the small intestine, which are brown and foul-smelling. This is known as *Faecal Vomiting*, although the vomited matter does not consist of formed faeces such as is present in the rectum.

There is *absolute constipation* which means that there is no passage of stools, but that no gas or flatus is passed either, even if an enema or suppository is given.

Distension of the abdomen is another important sign of intestinal obstruction

In some cases the patient may not appear to change much for some time even if not treated, but there will be a sudden collapse, and he will become extremely ill in a very short time. The obstruction may be caused by:

(a) A strangulated hernia.
(b) A large piece of food, or some swallowed body, or a gall-stone.
(c) Part of the intestine twisting on itself (volvulus) or kinking, or one part telescoping into another part. (Intussusception).
(d) Alteration of the wall of the intestine itself e.g. tumours, certain diseases.
(e) A band of fibrous tissue or adhesion round the outside of the intestine, or across it, pressing on it and preventing the passage of the contents.

When the obstruction is of the large bowel, the onset is usually more gradual. The patient may first complain of a feeling of fullness, i.e. distension. Sometimes there is difficulty in breathing because the distended bowel causes upward pressure on the heart and lungs. Pain and vomiting occur later in these cases, when the distended bowel allows the contents to pass back into the small intestine. There is nearly always a history of increasing constipation before the obstruction takes place. The cause of obstruction of the large bowel is often a growth, such as carcinoma (cancer), which gradually grows larger until it blocks the bowel.

Treatment: The patient is admitted to hospital. If he is in a state of collapse, measures are taken to improve his general condition before the operation is performed. A naso-gastric tube is passed into the stomach and the contents are aspirated completely. Nothing is given by mouth, but the body fluids and salts (sodium and potassium) which have been lost by vomiting are replaced by giving normal saline and other specially prepared solutions into a vein (intravenous 'drip'). An accurate intake/output fluid balance chart must be kept to ensure that the patient receives an adequate amount of fluid (2000–4000 ml per day) and that the urine output is satisfactory (about 1500 ml per day).

At operation the obstruction will be relieved, and it may be necessary to remove the damaged piece of intestine. The ends above and below are rejoined by stitches (intestinal anastomosis). In cases where there is a growth causing obstruction of the large intestine a colostomy (p. 22) is performed above the growth to allow the contents of the bowel to escape. The growth may be removed at another (second stage) operation and the colostomy closed by a third operation.

After the operation sips of water only are given at first, until some flatus has been passed, showing that the intestine is working. Gradually, a light diet is commenced, and this in increased as the patient improves.

In most non-urgent cases, drugs (e.g. phthalylsulphathiazole) are ordered to be given before and sometimes after the operation, to reduce the number of intestinal bacteria in order to prevent any infection which might complicate the operation.

J

Jaundice
Jaundice means an abnormal yellow colouring which can be seen most often in the skin and eyes. The colouring matter, which is called bilirubin, comes from the breakdown of the red blood cells, and in health it passes through the liver and colours the bile and causes the faeces to become brown. Jaundice therefore will occur as a result of:—

(1) Some kinds of anaemia when excessive numbers of red blood cells are being broken down too quickly (haemolytic anaemia).

(2) When the liver is damaged, as in inflammation (Hepatitis) caused by a virus, or when the liver is poisoned by some chemicals.

(3) In conditions where the bile, containing the colouring bilirubin, is not able to be excreted normally because of an obstruction of the bile ducts which run between the liver and the duodenum. Obstruction may be caused by such things as gall-stones.

In cases 2 and 3, the faeces are a greyish putty colour instead of being brown and the colouring matter appears in the urine which in its turn becomes brown. Testing will show the presence of bile in the urine.

K

Kidney Operations
Nephrectomy is the name given to the operation performed to remove the kidney. The operation may be necessary for a growth or a severe

chronic infection (pyelonephritis and tuberculosis). If the kidney is severely damaged by injury it may have to be removed to stop the haemorrhage which may threaten the patient's life.

Nephrostomy is the opening of the kidney to drain it, which may be done in an emergency when there is an obstruction to the passage of urine from the kidney and the patient is not well enough to have a more extensive operation carried out. It is usually carried out as a temporary measure until the patient's condition improves.

Nephrotomy or Nephro-lithotomy are the names given to the operations for opening the kidney, and the removal of stones. If the stones are in the pelvis of the kidney, the operation is known as *Pyelotomy or Pyelo-lithotomy*.

Tests of the function of the kidney are carried out before an operation. Most common are:

(1) *X-ray examination*, which shows up the presence of stones.

(2) *Cystoscopy*. A cystoscope is a long slender instrument with an internal light. This is passed into the bladder the inside of which can then be examined by the surgeon. One type of cystoscope allows a special catheter to be passed into the ureters, so that a separate specimen of urine may be obtained from each kidney.

(3) *Pyelography*. There are two types. The aim in each is to get an X-ray picture of the pelvis of the kidney after it has been filled with a special substance which shows up on the X-ray film:—

(*a*) *Intravenous or Excretion Pyelography (I.V.P.)* A substance (Hypaque) is injected into a vein, and passes through the circulation, to be excreted by the kidney. As it passes through the kidney, it shows up the renal pelvis and ureter. This injection is given when the patient is on the X-ray table, and films are taken at intervals every 5 or 10 minutes after it.

(*b*) *Retrograde or Instrumental Pyelography*. In this case a cystoscope is passed into the bladder, and a ureteric catheter is introduced into the ureter. The radio-opaque substance is then introduced directly into the pelvis of the kidney, and films are taken to show up the renal pelvis.

Preparation for any operation on the kidney is very similar. Abundant fluids are given and urinary antiseptics or other drugs will be ordered. An aperient is given 36 hours before operation, and an enema on the eve of the operation. A large area of skin is prepared depending on the site that the surgeon chooses to make his incision (loin or abdomen).

Usually an area of the trunk (lower chest and abdomen) is prepared from the axilla to the hip.

Post-operative care: As soon as the patient recovers from the effects of the anaesthetic he is sat up in bed, supported by pillows so that there is no strain on the wound. In many cases the surgeon places a drainage tube into the wound to allow the escape of urine or blood from the area. This may be removed after 48 hours or during the first week, depending on the amount of discharge. The patient may be supported, leaning towards the operated side to assist the drainage. The dressings must be changed as often as necessary, and this varies with the amount of drainage. If there is irritation the skin around the would may need the application of some protective cream or ointment.

The *amount of urine* passed must be measured and recorded, to enable the surgeon to judge the function of the kidney, especially after a nephrectomy when only one kidney remains.

Fluids are given by mouth as soon as the patient is able to take them. If necessary rectal fluids are ordered or intravenous fluids are given. *Diet* is started as soon as possible, and gradually increased. Drugs for the *relief of pain* will be required at first, and the surgeon often orders *antibiotic drugs* to prevent or overcome infection. An enema may be given after two days, if necessary.

If the wound is healing satisfactorily, the patient is allowed to get up towards the end of the first week, and he walks about for a few days before being discharged for convalescence.

L

Leukaemia

This is a disease of the tissues (reticulo-endothelial system, including the bone marrow, lymph nodes and spleen) which produce the white blood cells (leucocytes) which in Leukaemia are greatly increased in number. The cause is unknown. Any type of white cell may be affected the main ones being:

(i) The polymorphonuclear cells in Myeloid leukaemia
(ii) The lymphocytes in Lymphatic leukaemia
(iii) The monocytes in Monocytic leukaemia

Many immature cells appear in the blood.

It is normal for there to be an increase in the number of white cells following infection in the body, which is a reaction to help to overcome the bacteria or viruses which have invaded the body. This is known as leucocytosis. But leukaemia is a disease which is progressive and malignant. It may be acute, especially in children, and is then likely to be fatal after a few months. In older people it may be slower, and go on for several years with remissions (temporary abatement).

The patient suffers from loss of energy, and fatigue, and appears to be anaemic. The enormous number of white cells in the bone marrow upsets the normal formation of red cells and anaemia results. Purpura is commonly seen. In some cases the spleen and solidus or lymph nodes may be enlarged. The first symptom is often bleeding of ulcerated gums. A blood count is done to diagnose the condition if there is anaemia with enlarged lymph nodes and purpura. Usually a puncture is made into the sternum to withdraw some bone marrow to enable confirmation of the diagnosis.

Treatment: At present there is no known complete cure for leukaemia, but many drugs are now available which help to bring about long remissions. These can be ordered and changed as necessary, but may include prednisolone, Myleran, adriamycin, mercaptopurine. In some cases deep X-ray treatment or radio-active phosphorus may be used. Blood transfusions are also given.

Lung Operations

EMPYEMA. This refers to a collection of pus in between the two layers of the pleura surrounding the lungs. (This is a very thin double sheet of membrane which secretes a lubricating fluid and prevents friction as the lungs move on breathing). In most cases the condition is due to a spread of infection from the lung itself, but it may follow other septic conditions, such as an abscess under the diaphragm.

Chest Aspiration: If the pus is not too thick, and will run through a needle, it may be withdrawn (aspirated) by means of a syringe, and then an antibiotic drug is injected to kill the bacteria which are causing the formation of pus. So long as the pus remains fluid, these aspirations may be repeated with the injection of the antibiotic following, and this treatment may be sufficient to clear up the empyema.

Some bacteria produce a thick creamy pus which cannot be drawn through a needle, and in these cases an operation is performed to open the chest and clean out the area. This is known as *rib resection*. This operation is not often performed these days, as modern drugs are able to overcome the bacteria before the pus becomes thick. If it does become necessary to operate, the surgeon will open the chest wall over the empyema (removing a piece of rib) and he then opens the cavity. He cleans out the pus and fibrinous material that has accummulated, inserts a drainage tube, and closes the wound.

In some patients, whether treated by aspirations or by rib resection, the lung does not re-expand to fill the chest as it is encased by an inflamed and thickened layer of pleura. In order to get the lung to re-expand the surgeon has to peel off this thickened layer by an operation known as *decortication*.

Lobectomy: This is the removal of one lobe of a lung, and is most usually performed for tuberculosis, local bronchiectasis and occasionally for a cancer of the bronchus.

Pneumonectomy: This means the removal of a whole lung. The operation may be carried out in cases of carconima of the bronchus but it is only effective in early cases. After the operation the patient breathes with the remaining normal lung.

Segmental Resection means the removal of a segment or part of a lobe. This is mainly carried out for localised tuberculosis.

Pre-operative measures: If the operation is to be performed for tuberculosis, the patient will have had a long course of antituberculous drugs and his general condition improved as far as possible with good diet and general care. In cases of bronchiectasis, the patient is encouraged to expel as much sputum as possible, and postural drainage may be ordered.

POSTURAL DRAINAGE. The aim of postural drainage is to put the patient in such a position that the pus will drain naturally along the bronchus towards the trachea so that it will be coughed up and expelled. He is usually put to lie with the affected lung or part of the lung uppermost. For example, the foot of the bed is raised, so that the head is lower than the rest of the body, when the lower lobes are being drained. In some hospitals there are special beds for this purpose, which can be raised at the foot end by means of a handle, whilst the head of the bed is lowered. This drainage may be carried out daily, or in some cases three or four times a day. At the same time the physiotherapist will give breathing exercises and physical exercises. Sometimes the patient is sent to the country to have outdoor treatment in order to improve the general condition before being admitted to hospital for operation. If the operation is to be carried out for cancer, antibiotic drugs are usually given in order to reduce any infection. In all cases the blood is grouped and cross-matched, and all preparations are made for a blood transfusion.

Post-operative Care: On recovering from the anaesthetic, the patient will be propped up, well supported with pillows. He may be nursed with a humidifier to assist breathing. Oxygen will probably be required, and may be given through a comfortable mask. Blood transfusion is usually set up, and must be watched carefully. Fluids may be given by mouth as soon as the patient wishes. Pain and cough are eased by the administration of drugs. The rate of the pulse and respiration must be recorded regularly, and also the blood pressure. The patient is encouraged to cough, as it is extremely important that he expels the secretions. Drugs may be ordered to help to achieve this, and antibiotics are also given in most cases. Inhalations are sometimes used to help the patient to get rid of the sputum by coughing more easily.

DRAINAGE AFTER CHEST AND LUNG OPERATIONS. UNDERWATER-SEAL DRAIN

At the conclusion of a chest operation the surgeon inserts one or two drainage tubes (made of plastic material) into the pleural cavity in order that blood, serum and air will escape. If these tubes are allowed to drain into an ordinary container air will re-enter the pleural cavity each time the patient breathes in and the lung will not re-expand. It is necessary to have a kind of valve so that air can escape from the cavity but not re-enter. This valve is provided by the underwater seal bottle. Any air in the pleural cavity is blown out through the tubes and bubbles through the water during expiration or coughing and it cannot return into the chest providing that the tube from the patient's chest is always at least one inch below the level of the water.

Special care is needed when nursing a patient with an underwater-seal drain and nurses are strongly advised to make themselves thoroughly familiar with the procedures as taught to them in the classroom, on the wards and by the appropriate textbooks.

Lymphoma

This is a tumour composed of lymphatic tissue, of which there are many types. The cause is not known.

A simple benign tumour may be excised in most cases without any difficulty. There are other tumours which are not benign i.e. malignant. These may cause fever, sweating and loss of weight. Pressure on organs in the body cavities may be caused, if the lymph nodes in those areas are involved, resulting in signs and symptoms associated with those organs.

The condition can only be diagnosed by examination of some of the diseased tissue after it has been excised. The diagnosis and treatment are similar to that of Hodgkin's disease (p. 46).

M

Mastectomy

Mastectomy means removal of the breast. In a *simple mastectomy* only the breast and the covering skin are removed. A *radical mastectomy* is more extensive, for besides the breast and skin, the pectoral muscle (which lies under the breast) and the lymphatic tissue of the axilla are all removed.

Either kind of mastectomy may be carried out for cancer of the breast and for early cases a radical operation offers the best chance of cure, for cancer spreads very easily by the blood stream and the lymphatic system, as well as locally into the surrounding tissues.

A lump in the breast should never be ignored, and all women must be encouraged to seek medical advice immediately. The surgeon may advise the patient to have the lump removed and examined (frozen section biopsy) in the operating theatre. If it is a cancer it is better to perform the mastectomy straight away.

Pre-operatively: The patient is examined for the presence of spread of the cancer (secondary deposits or metastases). An X-ray of the chest is needed to exclude the presence of spread to the lungs. The blood is examined for the presence of anaemia. A pre-operative blood transfusion is required if anaemia is severe. Transfusion may also be given during the operation.

Skin Preparation: A large area of skin is prepared from the neck to the waist and from the opposite breast round the axilla (which must be shaved) and on as far as the spine. The arm, on the side of operation, down to the elbow will also be cleansed. A nurse may be surprised to learn that the thigh must also be washed and shaved before this operation. This is because a skin graft may be required, and this will probably be taken from the thigh. For this reason no strong antiseptics are applied on this area, as the cells on the surface of the skin would be damaged, and the skin will not graft so readily.

Post-operative Care: When the patient has recovered from the anaesthetic, she is sat up in bed, well supported, and a pillow may be put at the foot of the bed for her to push against and therefore to help her maintain her position. A blood transfusion or other intravenous fluid may be continued in case of shock. The nurse should ascertain the surgeon's wishes regarding the post-operative position of the arm on the operated side. Some surgeons bandage the arm to the side while others require it to be held away (abducted). A pillow is placed under the arm after the first day, and the patient is encouraged to carry out the movements which will be shown to her by the physiotherapist. She is taught how to move the arm gently and to gradually touch the back of her head, so that she will be able to dress herself and do her hair after her discharge from hospital.

The Wound: At least one tube is put into the wound at the operation because there is blood and serous fluid which must be allowed to escape. The dressing is packed when necessary; that is, when it becomes saturated. This is done by applying sterile dressings over the original dressing, and the bandage should be firmly applied. The dressing will not be changed for 24 to 48 hours, according to the surgeon's wishes. When it is changed, the tube will be gently eased and turned round, i.e. rotated. Any large amount of blood escaping into the dressing should be reported at once, before a packing is applied. The tube is removed when the drainage ceases, or in 2 to 4 days according to the instructions of the surgeon.

If a skin graft has been applied, great care will be required until it has become attached to the tissues underneath. In some cases stitches are used to prevent it being moved by the dressings, or by fluid collecting underneath it. Stitches in the wound are usually removed on the 8th to 12th day.

Fluids should be given freely as soon as possible after the operation and a normal diet gradually introduced. The patient may require some help with her meals until she regains the full use of the arm. She will be helped to get out of bed, into a chair, the day after the operation, and will be allowed up in 2 to 4 days. After the wound has healed satisfactorily, the patient should have at least two weeks' convalescence.

If she is worried at the thought of appearing "odd" or "one-sided" when dressed, it should be explained that an artificial breast can be made of cotton wool or foam rubber sponge, to enable the clothes to fit properly and to hide the disfigurement following the removal of the breast.

Radiotherapy and Follow-up: The surgeon usually arranges for the patient to have a course of radiotherapy as soon as the wound has healed. This lasts for about three weeks. Arrangements are made for the patient to visit the follow-up clinic at regular intervals after discharge.

Meningitis

This is inflammation of the meninges, which are the three coverings of the brain, and the spinal cord. Various types are described according to the organism which causes the inflammation, e.g. meningococcal, influenzal, pneumococcal, streptococcal, staphylococcal, tuberculous or viral.

The Signs and Symptoms are the same in all cases, due to the inflamed meninges causing pressure on the brain or cord. There are some special points about the different types, but in general:

The Onset is sudden (except in the tuberculous types) the patient being very ill with a high temperature and a relatively slow pulse. There is a persistent headache often associated with vomiting. The patient is irritable, drowsy, and may be delirious. His position in bed is typical; he lies curled up with his back to the light or window as he suffers from photophobia (dislike of light). In a child, there is a cry with a peculiarly high note, known as the "Meningeal cry", and convulsions or fits are common. A very typical sign in all cases is the rigidity of he neck muscles and it is difficult to flex the head.

Another sign that is seen is Kernig's sign:—With the thigh at right angles to the body, the patient is unable to straighten the leg at the knee, without pain. Special points are: i) In tuberculous Meningitis there is a gradual onset, often of 1 or 2 weeks, before the typical picture is seen. ii) Meningococcal Meningitis, the most common type, is also known as Cerebro-Spinal fever or Spotted Fever, because small spots may be found on the skin (Purpura, p. 79). It occurs in epidemics. iii) Pneumococcal and Influenzal Meningitis follow lung infections with these organisms as their names suggest. iv) Streptococcal and Staphylococcal Meningitis are caused by these bacteria usually following infection of the mastoid air cells of the skull (mastoiditis), a complication of infection of the middle ear (otitis media). The doctor will do a lumbar puncture to confirm the diagnosis, which will be suspected immediately from the condition of the patient. This is done with a completely aseptic technique, in order to obtain some of the cerebro-spinal fluid from between the layers of the meninges. A lumbar puncture needle is inserted between the lower lumbar vertebrae into the space between the two inner layers of the meninges (sub-arachnoid space). When the stilette is withdrawn the fluid drops out. After the first few drops, which may be bloodstained, have been allowed to run away, a sterile container is held to collect the fluid, and the pressure can be measured with a manometer. It is often possible to determine the exact type of meningitis by examination of this fluid.

Treatment: This very ill patient, who resents being disturbed, requires skilled and patient nursing, preferably in a quiet room to avoid disturbance, and with partly shaded light. Adequate fluids must be given with glucose at first, but after the appropriate drugs have had effect, a light diet may be given. Antibiotics and sulphonamide drugs enable the majority of patients to recover. There are special drugs to treat tuberculous meningitis, such as streptomycin, P.A.S. and isoniazid.

Migraine

This is a type of severe headache, with a feeling of sickness, and often the sight is disturbed, with "blurring", or seeing double (diplopia) or only half of what would normally be seen. These attacks usually start in teenagers, but become more severe, but less frequent, after middle age. An attack may last for many hours, and often ends with vomiting. The people who are sufferers from this condition, are often of highly-strung, and anxious temperaments, and do not seem able to relax. It is common for a busy person to work all the week, and then have an attack at the week-end, when she should be able to rest. There is some hereditary factor.

Treatment: Prevention of overstrain, relaxation regularly, and holidays if possible, will help to prevent attacks.

The doctor may order drugs, which are given for several months, to try to prevent the attacks, by calming the patient, and soothing the nerves e.g. ergotamine.

During an attack, drugs may be ordered for the relief of pain.

Myxoedema

This condition arises when the thyroid gland, at the front of the neck does not form enough or any of its secretion. In a baby, it causes cretinism, when the baby does not grow normally, either mentally or physically.

In an adult, who has already grown, the gland may stop its usual secretion either through disease, or removal of the gland. It is most commonly seen in women.

All the functions of the body become slowed mentally and physically, the eyelids are puffy, and the face is without any expression, and the skin has a yellowish appearance, but with a patch of red on each cheek. The hands and feet are puffy. The speech becomes slow, and the patient gradually becomes mentally slow, with a poor memory. This is all due to the fact that the secretion from the thyroid gland controls the rate at which the food is used up by the body, and when the secretion is missing, the rate becomes so slow, that all bodily functions are slow, too.

Treatment: Special tablets are given to the patient containing thyroid extract for the rest of her life, and the condition soon clears up, the patient regaining her normal appearance and mental ability.

N

Nephritis

Nephritis is also known as Bright's disease, from a doctor of that name, who described it.

Nephritis in inflammation of the kidney, and it may follow some infection such as tonsillitis, scarlet fever or pneumonia.

The patient: There may be a sudden onset of the illness, with a raised temperature, vomiting, swelling of the eyelids and face, and very little urine is passed, and this may be blood stained. In a milder case, no blood is seen, but when the urine is tested, it is found to contain albumen.

As the nephritis becomes more severe, the oedema spreads all over the body. The amount of urine passed becomes less and less and, if blood is present it looks to be a reddish brown colour, or even blood coloured.

With treatment, the condition of the patient gradually improves, but a trace of albumen may be found in the urine for some time. If there is no permanent damage to the kidneys, this will gradually clear up, altogether.

Some of these cases do not recover, but the nephritis becomes chronic. This is only in about 10% to 15% of cases.

Treatment: Rest for the patient and for the kidneys is very important, and this must be continued until blood has disappeared from the urine. There are no special drugs to cure this condition. The patient should be kept warm, and away from draughts. Fluid restriction is important at first, and a fluid Intake and Output chart must be carefully kept. Specimens of urine will be required each day, for testing.

The fluids will probably be restricted to 2 pints of fruit drinks, with extra glucose, and this will be kept up until the oedema disappears. At the same time, salt will be cut down in the diet, even when the fluid intake is increased, as the output of urine increases.

Drugs may be ordered for any infection in the body, such as inflamed tonsils.

The heart may be affected by the strain in nephritis, and careful watch is kept on the pulse rate.

Severe headache or convulsions may be caused by the oedema in the brain, and drugs are ordered to relieve this.

CHRONIC NEPHRITIS

This may be the result of any disease of the kidney, and it may also be seen in patients who have a long-standing high blood pressure. The kidney develops renal failure, in some instances, with increasing oedema. There is anaemia, the patient has a pale muddy complexion, and often, he complains of digestive disturbances, such as hiccups, diarrhoea, and vomiting. Then the condition known as Uraemia develops, which means that poisonous substances are accumulating in the blood, instead of being excreted.

CHRONIC RENAL FAILURE

The amount of urine that is excreted increases, and it is very dilute and pale in colour. The patient often has to get up in the night to pass urine, and so his sleep is disturbed. Every system of the body is affected:

Nervous System: The patient feels tired and without energy, and if not treated, will become drowsy, and this may go on until he is in a uraemic coma, that is, a state of deep unconsciousness. His muscles may twitch, and he may have fits, similar to the ones seen in epilepsy.

Digestive System: The breath smells of urine, the tongue is dry, and brown in colour, and the patient feels sick, and may vomit.

Respiratory System: Deep sighing breathing is often seen, and later the breathing may become irregular, from a period almost without breathing, short shallow breaths are taken, and these become quicker and deeper, and then decrease again, to a period when breathing seems to stop. This is known as Cheyne-Stokes breathing, and is usually a danger signal, and means that the patient is extremely ill.

Heart and Blood Vessels: Because there is usually high blood pressure with this condition, the heart may show signs of failing, or there may be a haemorrhage from a blood vessel, but the most common cause of death, in this condition, is failure of the kidneys, themselves. Some anaemia is always present.

The Skin: Because the sweat glands are doing extra work, excreting some of the substances which the kidneys should excrete, the skin is irritated, and there is a general itchiness of the skin known as pruritis. It is dry, and rather yellow in colour.

Treatment: Drugs are given to relieve the high blood pressure. The patient may be ordered a strict diet, but this is not so common now, as it is considered more important to keep the patient comfortable, and without distress, as nothing can be done to prevent the kidneys from failing, in the end.

CHRONIC NEPHRITIS—URAEMIA

If there is no sign of heart failure, a blood transfusion may be given for the anaemia slowly, with some benefit.

The nursing care of the patient with this condition entails looking after the comfort and peace of mind, as well as the routine procedures, more carefully than in many cases.

If a special diet is ordered, it usually is one with a low amount of proteins, (i.e. decreased meat, fish, eggs, cheese, etc.) but he can have other foods as he wishes. In some cases, the amount of salt is also regulated.

O

Oedema

This is a collection of excess fluid in the tissues, due to one or several causes:

(i) In heart failure. This is because (a) the heart does not cope adequately with the blood returning from the whole of the body via, the two great veins, the inferior and superior vena cavae. The backpressure builds up, and fluid is forced from the vessels into the tissues; (b) the kidneys are not able to excrete waste products, especially salt, from the body and so water is retained to maintain the correct concentration of salt in the tissues.
(ii) Chronic Nephritis.
(iii) Venous obstruction e.g. Thrombosis.
(iv) A tumour (e.g. a cancer) which causes pressure on veins, particularly in the pelvis, oedema being seen in the legs.

The nurse can distinguish oedema from other swelling by pressing lightly with a finger on the area. A "pit" is formed which remains for some time after the finger is lifted. The nurse will often see the doctor carry out this test. The treatment will be for the condition which is caused the oedema.

P

Paralysis

This is the loss of the power of movement of some part of the body, due to disease or injury of the nervous system. There are two types of paralysis, depending on where the damage to the nerves of the muscles, has occured. It may be that the muscle remains fixed and rigid, known as spastic, or the muscle may be flabby and limp, and this is known as flaccid (pronounced *flaksid*). In this latter type, the muscles are liable to waste away. Different names are used to describe the amount of paralysis:

Monoplegia—means one limb is paralysed.

Hemiplegia—means that the whole of one side of the body is paralysed, (which signifies that the damage to the nerves is in the brain, which controls them). Paraplegia--the name given when the lower half of the body is paralysed, (and signifies that the damage is in the spinal cord). In this case, there is no control over the bladder or bowel, generally, and so the patient will be incontinent.

The above types of paralysis all refer to the motor nerves in the body, i.e. controlling movement.

If the nerves which are damaged are those which carry sensations into the brain, or that part of the brain that receives them is damaged, then the sensations or feelings of the patient will be disturbed. Sometimes, both the motor and sensory nerves are damaged, and so, with paralysis of the muscles there may be:

(a) Loss of sensation—known as anaesthesia. In a paralysed patient this may be very dangerous, as he will not feel a burn, for example.
(b) Increased feeling in an area—known as Hyperaesthesia.
(c) Unusual sensations—known as paraesthesia e.g., "pins and needles", tingling, etc.

At the same time, there may be loss of speech, sight, hearing, taste or smell.

Nursing: After the injury to the nerves, there may be improvement in the condition of the patient, for some time, and there may be complete recovery.

In nursing a paralysed patient, the pressure areas require special care. If the control of the muscles at the openings of the bladder and rectum is lost, the nurse must realise that she will be expected to help the patient over this difficulty. Often, with training, the bladder will be emptied quite regularly, but, in the first stages, catheterising will probably be necessary. The danger of infection must always be remembered in this condition.

If the patient is not able to move about, and lies still in bed, there is a danger of the fluid in the lungs (which is normally coughed out) becoming stagnant, and infected. There is therefore, a great danger of pneumonia developing. This is known as Hypostatic Pneumonia (static means still), and a complication to be avoided by all possible means. This type of pneumonia is liable to develop in any patient who remains still for a long time.

The position of the patient is changed every two hours, to try to prevent this. Pressure areas may be protected by air cushions, foam rubber mattresses, etc.

The mental outlook of the patient is almost as important as his physical condition, and he has to be encouraged to realise that life can go on, and he can be a useful member of society, even though paralysed.

Paralytic Ileus

Paralysis of the bowel which is known as paralytic ileus may occur from peritonitis or after abdominal operations when the intestine has been exposed, manipulated or become infected. Because of the paralysis and lack of movement, the intestine becomes dilated, and the contents regurgitate into the stomach (regurgitate means to pass backwards in the wrong direction). There may be little pain, but distension, constipation and vomiting are the usual signs. If a stethoscope is placed on the abdomen it will be found that the bowel sounds have disappeared. The pulse rate is increased, and the patient looks ill.

The Treatment: This aims at resting the paralysed intestine, and emptying the stomach by a naso-gastric tube at regular intervals. A flatus tube may be ordered to be passed into the rectum and the surgeon may request this to be repeated 4-hourly. Intravenous fluids will be given, and a record is kept of the fluid intake and output. Small amounts of fluid are sometimes given by mouth (if the patient asks for a drink) as it will be syphoned back when the stomach is next aspirated. Antibiotic drugs may be ordered when peritonitis is the cause. Drugs for the relief of pain and discomfort may also be required. The paralysis is quickly overcome in most cases, and the nurse should note and report if any flatus is passed as this is one of the first signs of recovery.

During the treatment for this condition, the hygiene of the mouth is very important, and requires regular attention. Pieces of pineapple or orange may be given for the patient to chew and spit out, or chewing gum may be used if the patient is well enough. These acid fruits help to encourage the flow of saliva and prevent infection of the parotid salivary glands (parotitis) which is a very painful complication.

Peptic Ulcer (see p. 93).

Phimosis

This is the condition which calls for the operation known as *circumcision* (which means cutting round). The foreskin or prepuce at the end of the penis is too small or tight, and cannot be drawn back as it should normally. It may therefore interfere with the passage of urine, and the area underneath is liable to become infected, as it cannot be cleaned, so causing Balanitis—or inflammation of the glans penis. It may occur in young children, or adults, due to repeated attacks of balanitis, and it happens very occasionally in young or newly born babies. At circumcision the foreskin is cut away, and the remaining edges of skin and mucous membrane are stitched together with fine catgut. After the operation the wound must be kept clean, especially after the passing of urine (micturition). Antiseptic dressings are applied around the end of the penis, or boracic fomentations may be applied, and changed after micturition. If the patient is not admitted to hospital, a dressing soaked in Tincture of Benzoin (Friar's Balsam) may be applied, left for 5 to 6 days, and then be soaked off in a warm bath. The stitches (Catgut or Dexon) will fall out without further attention.

Pilonidal Sinus

This is a blind track or space containing a nest of hairs which forms in the cleft between the buttocks. It is common in well covered hairy young men and women, and is related to occupations or pastimes involving a lot of sitting (particularly including lorry driving, rowing etc.) Often infected, recurrent abscesses may form. Rarely, the track is congential from birth and leads down to the spine. This type is not truly a pilonidal sinus.

Treatment: The treatment is surgical. The area is cleaned and shaved. All visible tracks are properly excised. If an abscess has formed it will be incised. Removal of the sinus may be performed later. The area around is shaved and kept free of hair after the operation. The patient may be nursed lying on the side or prone.

Pneumoconiosis

This is a chronic condition of the lungs, caused by the inhalation of dust. The reaction to this irritation is the formation of fibrous tissue, as in any other case of chronic irritation such as tuberculosis and bronchiectasis.

Pneumoconiosis is also known as the "dust disease" and is most commonly seen as:

(i) Silicosis in stone workers, gold miners, potters.
(ii) Asbestosis in asbestos workers.
(iii) Anthracosis in anthracite coal miners.
(iv) Siderosis in steel workers, also in tin miners and lead miners.
(v) Calciocosis in marble workers.

This is known as an occupational hazard, as there is always the danger of developing the disease in these occupations.

The patient becomes short of breath (i.e. dyspnoeic), with a chronic cough and sputum. An X-ray examination will show a typical picture of the lungs, with the fibrous tissue showing up throughout the lungs as "blotchy" areas. One of the dangers is the possibility of tuberculosis invading the lungs. When the condition is diagnosed the patient must change his work, preferably to an open air job, otherwise the condition will progress, leading to eventual heart failure.

Prevention is an important aspect. The atmosphere at the works should be kept damp, and extractor fans may be used to draw out the dust from the air. Respirators should be worn when possible.

Pneumonia

Pneumonia is inflammation of the lung, caused by bacteria. The inflammation causes swelling of the lung in the infected area, which becomes solid, instead of remaining soft and spongy. The breathing is hampered as air cannot get into the air spaces in the solid part.

Lobar Pneumonia is an infection, usually in a part of one lung only, caused by a particular bacterium—the pneumococcus. The parts of the lung are called lobes, hence the name—lobar.

Broncho-pneumonia is more common and is caused by various kinds of bacteria (e.g. staphylococcus). The smaller bronchial tubes are affected and the condition tends to be patchy in both lungs.

The Patient: The illness may begin suddenly, often with a violent attack of shivering (Rigor p. 85). The temperature rises quickly to 103°—104° F, the pulse rate is increased, there is pain in the chest, and a dry cough. The patient complains of feeling ill, he has a headache, and may feel sick, and actually vomit.

Treatment: An antibiotic drug will be ordered at the onset, as soon as the doctor diagnoses Pneumonia. The cause of the illness can often be found from a specimen of sputum, or of blood. When the germ has been identified, the drug which is most active against that particular bacterium will be used. This is usually sufficient to stop the infection, and the temperature becomes normal in 2 to 3 days, but the area in the lung that has been infected will take some time to return to normal.

Oxygen may be administered in the early stages, if the breathing is distressed, or if the patient is blue (cyanosed).

As rest and sleep are important, drugs may be ordered to be given at night. A poultice e.g., kaolin, may be applied to the painful side of the chest. Antibiotics are used.

The patient is nursed sitting up, supported by pillows, and is disturbed as little as possible. A cough mixture may be ordered. The diet should be normal, as far as possible, with extra fluids. If the patient does not wish to eat, extra fluids with sugar or glucose are encouraged.

Pneumothorax

This is a collection of air between the two layers of pleura, which cover the lungs and lines the inside of the chest wall. It may occur from a penetrating wound of the chest, by rupture of an abscess or cavity of the lung, or of an air sac or bronchiole. A spontaneous pneumothorax is a pneumothorax occurring suddenly without any obvious reason but is usually found to be due to rupture of an air sac (alveolus) in cases of emphysema (p. 84) Pneumothorax has a sudden onset with severe pain on the affected side of the chest, and breathlessness. If a large amount of air is present the lung collapses, with severe dyspnoea and cyanosis (blueness of the skin). Clinical examination by the doctor and X-rays will confirm the diagnosis.

Treatment: In most cases the air will soon be absorbed if the patient rests in bed, and the lung will then expand. If there is severe dyspnoea and cyanosis some of the air must be removed to relieve the tension. The doctor puts a needle between the ribs into the air in the cavity, and a long rubber tube attached to it. The other end of this tube is put into a bottle of water, allowing the air to bubble out through it, but air is not able to re-enter (under-water seal). If the ruptured lung does not heal, the surgeon will have to operate.

Prostatectomy

The prostate gland lies at the base of the urinary bladder in the male, and the urethra passes through it. This means that the urine has to pass down through the urethra (or duct) which is inside the gland. If the gland becomes enlarged or swollen the flow of urine may be interfered with. The urine would then accumulate in the bladder, and eventually become full and cause back pressure up the ureters. The ureters are the ducts which carry the urine from the kidneys, so therefore the kidneys them selvesmay then be affected and they may begin to fail. An enlarged prostate gland must be treated as soon as possible, or the life of the patient may be in danger.

Symptoms and signs. An enlarged prostate is fairly common in men over 50 years of age. It is often a simple enlargement, but it may be due to carcinoma. The patient will complain of difficulty of micturition. He has difficulty in starting to pass urine, and only a small amount may be passed each time. The patient will have disturbed nights, and loss of sleep, as he will have to get up two or more times to pass a small amount of urine each time (frequency). The urine may be blood-stained (haematuria) as a result of congestion of the base of the bladder. He will often complain of pain and a scalding sensation on micturition, which is due to infection in the stagnant urine. The patient may have retention of urine, and is either not able to pass any urine (acute retention) or the bladder is full and the urine overflows in small amounts (retention with overflow). If retention is neglected the patient may become drowsy, complain of headache, develop twitchings of the muscles, and finally become unconscious (in a coma) from uraemia (Uraemic Coma).

Simple enlargement of the prostate is treated by prostatectomy. If the enlargement is due to carcinoma, certain drugs (e.g. Stilboestrol) may be ordered which are found to reduce the size of the organ.

In preparation for the operation the patient is made as well as possible. Any infection of the urine is treated and he is encouraged to drink large quantities of fluids. A fluid intake and output chart is always necessary. The blood is examined to find out if anaemia is present and also to measure the amount of urea in the blood (blood urea) as this will be increased if the kidneys are not functioning properly. Other investigations of the functions of the kidneys include various chemical tests (creatinine clearance) and X-rays (Intravenous Pyelogram p. 80). The operation most usually carried out nowadays is one in which the surgeon operates through the wall of the lower abdomen just behind the pubic bones. This is called a retropubic prostratectomy. When the patient returns to the ward, he may have two tubes, one in the incision to drain the wound and the other (a catheter) in the urethra to drain the bladder.

Post-operatively: The immediate risks are heamorrhage and shock. The patient should be protected from cold and propped up as soon as he regains consciousness if his condition permits. Fluids may be given intravenously for the first 24 to 48 hours, and he should be encouraged to drink as much as possible to keep the kidneys acting. A fluid intake and output chart must be accurately recorded, as, if necessary, more fluids will have to be given intravenously. The pulse should be recorded half-hourly to begin with, as the rate will increase if haemorrhage occurs.

The tube in the wound is usually removed after two days and the wound allowed to heal. The catheter will be allowed to drain into a special type of plastic bag, and this should be watched. If there appears to be an increase in the amount of blood in the urine or the tube becomes blocked by blood clot this fact should be reported. Some surgeons order a bladder wash-out to be given at regular intervals. This may be with normal saline, plain water, or a solution of sodium citrate. This is carried out through the catheter which is already in position. Antibiotics or similar drugs are usually ordered for five to seven days after the operation to overcome any infection.

A sorbo rubber or air bed is often used as this will not absorb any urine or blood which might leak into the bed. The bed, must, however, be kept dry, and the pressure areas are treated frequently. The patient is encouraged to move about the bed to prevent chest complications and thrombosis (clotting) in the veins of the legs. Fluids by mouth are maintained and a light diet is given as soon as the patient wishes, and gradually increased to a normal diet. The second day after the operation he may be allowed to get up with the surgeon's permission, and then allowed up for longer periods, if all goes well.

Protrusion of an Intervertebral Disc   (Slipped Disc)

Between the vertebrae (bones of the spine), there are discs which allow the movement of the whole spine. If one (or more) of these discs protrudes, i.e. juts out from its normal position, it will press on the first part of spinal nerves in the area (known as the nerve root). These nerves come from the spinal cord, which is inside the vertebrae, to supply the trunk and limbs. If there is pressure on a nerve root, there is usually acute pain.

The most common site for this to occur is in the lumbar region and the resulting pain is in the back and leg, and is often thought to be lumbago or sciatica. The "slipped disc" may be caused by lifting heavy articles, using the wrong muscles, and so straining the back. The pain may be very sudden in onset, and when the patient bends down he is unable to straighten up again. On the other hand, if the disc gradually protrudes more and more, the pain will not be so severe at first but will increase as the bulge of the disc increases. Depending on the nerves affected there may be feelings of numbness or tingling.

Treatment: Complete rest in bed, on a mattress which is kept level, for which fracture boards are useful. Drugs may be ordered to relieve the pain. Traction of the legs (skin traction) may be applied as it stretches the spine, prevents movement, and often gives relief. The physiotherapist will visit the patient regularly, and give him exercises to maintain the tone of the muscles of the back.

Some surgeons prefer to apply a plaster jacket round the part of the spine, to support and rest it. In this case, the patient will be able to carry on with his normal life, except that he is warned not to lift heavy weights. The jacket may be worn for 8 to 12 weeks, even though the pain will have almost disappeared in a few days. After the plaster is removed, the surgeon may order a special type of supporting corset to be worn for several months. This is strengthened with metal bars and prevents strain on the spine. If these measures do not cure the condition, it may be necessary to operate, especially if there are repeated attacks of severe pain. The operation commences with a laminectomy, which is the removal of parts of the laminae of the vertebrae. (The lamina of a vertebra is the piece of bone which passes out sideways from the central body). This is done so that the surgeon can reach the discs and remove the part that has "slipped" i.e. the protruding part which is causing the pressure.

After operation the patient is nursed lying flat on the back for one or two days. Some surgeons allow him to lie on the side opposite to the one on which the operation was carried out. The length of time that the patient remains in bed will be decided by the surgeon, but it is usually between 12 and 21 days. Physiotherapy will be started soon after the patient is comfortable after the operation, that is to say in about 3 days. Occupational therapy is also useful.

Purpura

This is a condition in which haemorrhages occur into the skin, mucous membrane, serous membrane or elsewhere. In the skin, purpura causes purple spots, known as *Petechiae* if very small, and as *Macules* if larger spots. Large patches may also be formed. There are many conditions which may cause purpura such as:

(i) Purpura Simplex (or Senile Purpura) the most common kind, is found in older people. The spots come and go but do not affect the health and are not considered important.

(ii) Diminished Platelets (thrombocytes) in the blood, causing Thrombocytopenic or Haemorrhagic Purpura. This occurs in diseases of the bone marrow, where the platelets are made, or of the blood itself as in Leukaemia where the platelets are lacking in numbers, due to the excess white cells.

(iii) Damaged blood vessel walls as in infectious illnesses such as Meningococcal Meningitis, severe scarlet fever, measles, smallpox, and in other conditions where bacteria invade the body, and in some cases of arthritis.

(iv) Some drugs such as cortisone, sulphonamides and even aspirin may cause purpura. Deficiency of Vitamin C (found in many foods normally) may also result in Purpura. Both are known as Secondary Purpura.

(v) Allergy. In a condition of "nettle rash" (urticaria) there may be some purpura, also after taking some foods to which the patient is hypersensitive or allergic.

Treatment: This depends on the cause, which will be diagnosed as soon as possible, and the appropriate drugs and nursing care will be prescribed.

Pyelitis and Pyelo-Nephritis

Pyelitis means inflammation of the pelvis of the kidney, which is the hollow part connected to the ureter. It collects the urine from the kidney, to pass it along to the ureter and so to the bladder.

This is more commonly seen in women than in men, and is often caused by the bacteria which normally live in the bowel. When they get into the urinary tract, they cause inflammation because this tract is normally sterile.

When the pelvis of the kidney is infected, there is always some damage to the kidney substance itself so the name of Pyelo-Nephritis is commonly used to include both.

If there are frequent attacks of infection the kidneys may eventually fail to function and this is extremely serious.

The Patient: There is a sudden onset with the patient feeling ill, having shivering attacks (rigors), aching in the lower part of the back on one or both sides, and the temperature rises rapidly to 102°—103° F. and remains high. The tongue is coated, the pulse faster than normal, and there may be constipation, or vomiting. The urine looks cloudy, and is passed frequently, causing scalding pain to the patient.

Treatment: Rest in bed is essential until the temperature is normal and the acute urinary symptoms have been eased. The patient should drink at least 5 to 6 pints of fluids per day, and a record of the intake and output must be made carefully. Drugs will be ordered, and these may be changed when the doctor has received the report from the laboratory informing him what organisms are present in the urine, and which drugs will be the most useful. To ensure rest at night sedative drugs may also be ordered. After 3 or 4 days of treatment, the signs and symptoms will usually have disappeared, unless some unusual germ is the cause. In any case, a complete investigation of the urinary tract will probably be carried out, to try to see if there is any obstruction or other cause for the infection developing. If urine is allowed to remain stationary (stagnant) in any part of the tract it may become infected by bacteria. Tests may include X-ray examinations, cystoscopy, ureteric catheterisation, pyelography.

As a patient is liable to have further attacks of pyelitis after the first infection, her resistance should be built up with a good nourishing diet and fresh air. Exercise is important but she should avoid becoming over-tired.

Pyloric Stenosis

The pylorus is the lower end of the stomach, where there is a muscle surrounding the opening through which food passes into the duodenum and on into the intestine. 'Stenosis' means narrowing. Pyloric Stenosis therefore, is narrowing of the pyloric end of the stomach. This may be seen in babies, usually male babies, who are otherwise healthy. It may also be seen in patients who have had ulceration of the stomach or duodenum near the pylorus. As healing of an ulcer takes place scar tissue forms and this tends to shrink and may lead to stenosis (see p. 86).

In a baby, the muscle which surrounds the pylorus overgrows or increases in size (hypertrophy) more than is normal. This causes thickening and results in narrowing of the opening, and the condition is known as *Congenital Hypertrophic Pyloric Stenosis*. The baby is healthy and seems to be doing well for the first two or three weeks, but then he starts to vomit and his condition rapidly deteriorates. The vomiting occurs suddenly after a feed and the returned milk shoots out forcibly, extending perhaps two or three feet from the baby. This is known as projectile vomiting. This loss of food and fluid from the body can be very serious, particularly in such a young baby. The baby loses weight quickly, and soon looks very ill, unless treatment is given.

Treatment of Pyloric Stenosis in a baby: In a mild case, drugs may be given to prevent the closing or spasm of the muscle. Now, however in most cases an operation, known as Ramstedt's operation is very successful. Subcutaneous infusions of saline are ordered to correct the loss of fluid (dehydration), and the stomach is washed out daily in preparation for the operation. The baby must be kept warm, and may be wrapped in cotton wool, or in woollen clothes, with only the abdomen exposed at the operation. The operation is carried out as quickly as possible, to avoid the loss of body heat. A general or local anaesthetic is given, the abdomen is opened and the surgeon divides the thickened muscle which is closing the pylorus.

Post-operatively the baby is either nursed lying flat or is propped up in a little chair ('Echo' chair), and the administration of fluid subcutaneously is continued. The temperature is taken each hour, for 6 to 12 hours, according to instructions. If a temperature of 100° F. is reached the woollen clothing is removed, and, if there is still a raised temperature a tepid sponging may be ordered.

Feeding the baby after the operation varies according to the wishes of the surgeon. In some cases, a small feed of glucose (from 1 to 4 teaspoonfuls) may be given two hours after the return from the theatre, but some surgeons may order breast milk to be given if the baby is breast-fed normally. The feed is increased in amount and frequency until by the 3rd or 4th day a diet suitable for a child of the same age and weight is being given, if there is no vomiting or diarrhoea. If either of these should occur it should be reported immediately. A careful check is kept on the weight of the baby, as a gradual increase shows that satisfactory progress is being made.

The infant is sent home as soon as possible, to prevent the danger of infection from other cases in the hospital. He may be allowed to go home on the 4th day, and return to have the stitches removed from the abdominal wound on the 7th or 8th day.

R

Raynaud's Disease and Sympathectomy

The Automatic Nervous System supplies the blood vessels with nerves which carry the impulses to expand and contract these vessels as required. Part of this system, known as the sympathetic chain, lies in front of the spine, one chain on each side of the vertebral column. In Raynaud's Disease exposure of hands or feet to cold makes the blood vessels go into spasm (contract tightly) so that the flow of blood is impeded. The fingers feel dead and go white or a dusky blue, and on rewarming they go a red colour. This disease affects the upper limbs most often, and it is seen more often in women than in men. If the condition is severe and continuous the affected part may die from lack of oxygen (which the blood carries to the cells) and gangrene will follow.

The treatment for a severe case of Raynaud's disease is sympathectomy. This operation consists of removal of parts of the nerve tissue in the sympathetic chain, on each side. As the condition usually occurs on both sides of the body (e.g. the fingers of both hands most commonly), both sides may be operated upon at the same time. A cervical sympathectomy is carried out for Raynaud's disease affecting the hands. The operation is carried out through an opening made in the neck near the clavicle, in the axilla, or beside the scapula. If the lower limbs are affected, a lumbar sympathectomy is carried out. In this case the incision may be made in the lumbar region of the back, or through the abdomen.

After the operation, which is not a very serious one, there are complications which the nurse should watch for and report. There may be swelling and bruising locally (haematoma). The patient may complain of burning pains in the part of the body near to the incision. These may be present for a few weeks but will gradually diminish.

If the chest has been opened to perform the operation for the relief of Raynaud's disease of the hands there may be chest complications, such as complaints of difficulty in breathing. The surgeon will order X-ray pictures to be taken, to ascertain if air or fluid has entered the pleural cavity, and it is likely that the chest will be drained and the tube connected to an underwater seal bottle (p. 76).

Rheumatism (Acute) or Rheumatic Fever

There are several types of Rheumatism. It was often thought to be associated with poor housing, and is common in this country, and in most places where there is a climate similar to ours. In many cases it follows infections such as sore throat or tonsillitis, therefore it is thought that it may be the reaction of the body to the germ which causes these. Usually it is seen in young people, between 5 and 15 years.

The Patient: Usually, the illness starts rather suddenly, maybe some 2–3 weeks after a sore throat. There is a raised temperature (100°–101° F.) but may be much higher, with a general feeling of being "off-colour". The appetite is lost, the tongue is furred and there may be constipation. The patient complains of pains in the joints, which moves (flits) from one joint to another at different times. Some of the joints become swollen, and then subside, as another joint is affected. The affected joints may be hot and tender to touch. This condition requires early treatment, to avoid serious complications. The joint pains are not to be dismissed as mere growing pains.

Treatment: Rest. Pulse rate. Exercises. Rest in bed, with no exertion, is one of the most important points in treating acute rheumatism, therefore the nursing must be carried out very carefully. There is danger of the heart being damaged by the poisonous substances which circulate in the blood stream from this infection. The patient is not allowed to do anything for himself until all signs of the disease have disappeared. Exercise is gradually allowed so long as there is no increase in the pulse rate. This must be carefully noted, and the sleeping pulse is often used as a guide (taken whilst the patient is asleep.) This is better indication than the waking pulse, which may remain higher than normal for some time. If the sleeping pulse becomes slower the condition of the patient is improving. Long term penicillin is given after initial high dosage.

Position in bed: The patient is nursed in the most comfortable position, and the painful joints may be supported on pillows, or by splints or bandages, over cotton wool, to prevent any movement which causes pain. A cradle is used in the bed, to take the weight of the bed clothes.

Tepid sponging, and changing the clothes and sheets may be necessary once or twice each day if there is much sweating. As much fluid is lost from the body in this way, the patient is encouraged to drink extra fluids. As soon as she feels able to eat a good diet should be given.

Sedimentation Rate (E.S.R.) measurements are carried out at intervals, as when this reaches normal, it will show that the activity of the disease has come to an end.

Drugs will be ordered to relieve the pain and reduce the severity of the illness, but they do not cure the rheumatism. Penicillin may also be ordered, not for the rheumatism, but for any infection, such as sore throat, which may produce the condition.

Convalescence must be allowed, for quite a period, and at the seaside or in the country if possible.

If the temperature remains high, with a rapid pulse rate and often with pain in the chest, it is a sign that the disease is spreading. It may spread to the nerve tissue in the brain, and this will be shown by jerky, uncontrolled movements, and this is known as St. Vitus Dance or Chorea.

Rib Fracture

This condition is frequently seen these days as the ribs can be fractured by crushing, e.g. in a motor accident. There is severe pain over the area made worse by breathing. The lung underneath may be torn and air gets into the subcutaneous tissues (surgical emphysema) causing an area which is swollen and "crackles" on touching. If the air gets into the pleural cavity, it is known as Pneumothorax. If there are multiple fractures, the chest will become unstable (flail chest) and the casualty cannot ventilate his lungs properly, and it follows that the owygenation of the blood is reduced (anoxia) which in turn affects the function of the heart and the brain.

Treatment of the fracture aims at relieving the pain and preventing pulmonary complications. In mild cases the patient may be kept in bed for 24 hours and a local anaesthetic such as novocain may be injected. The ribs unite easily, and occasionally are strapped with 3-inch strapping, applied round the affected side, from the spine to the sternum, starting well below the injury and continuing to overlap the previous strapping to above the fracture. After the first shock is over, the patient is encouraged to get up and move about, to prevent complications such as pneumonia, especially in elderly people. Antibiotics may be ordered prophylactically (preventatively).

In cases of multiple fractures, intensive care is necessary and the patient may require either an intratracheal tube or a tracheostomy so

that proper ventilation of the lungs, and therefore oxygenation of the blood, be achieved by a mechanical ventilator (e.g. Cape).
Haemothorax may follow fractured ribs.

Rigor

This is the name given to an attack of shivering, with a rapid rise of temperature, often seen at the beginning of an infectious fever. It is the reaction of the body to the foreign substances (toxins) from the germs which enter the blood stream. It may also occur when a foreign protein is injected into the body. Although the temperature is rising, the patient feels cold. In 15 to 30 minutes, the patient complains of feeling very hot, and the skin is hot and dry. After about 1 hour or longer, there is profuse sweating, and the temperature falls to normal.

Nursing: During the shivering stage, the patient may be given an extra blanket, and a well covered hot water bottle, outside the blanket, at the feet. When the hot stage starts these may be removed. The nurse should note the length of time that the rigor lasts and also the temperature, and these should be reported. After the attack is over, the patient should be made comfortable, and allowed to rest. If, during the rigor, the patient is nervous and seems worried about his condition, the nurse may explain that it is the body, fighting the infection, that is causing the heat and shivering. A rigor is not common in children, except in cases of scarlet fever, and disease of the kidney.

S

Sarcoidosis

This is a disease of unknown origin which affects young adults and sometimes older people (20–40 years). It is characterised by lesions resembling tuberculosis, but no tubercule bacilli are found. Periods of activity are followed by periods of recovery. The lesions may affect:
    (i) The skin—causing pink nodules on the face and chest, and there may be painful red areas on the shins and forearms, often the first sign.

(ii) The lungs—causing dyspnoea and cough. X-ray pictures show patches in the lungs.
(iii) Lymph nodes—causing swollen nodes (glands) in the neck and chest. The salivary glands in the mouth may also be affected.
(iv) The bones—in the extremities. Excess calcium appears in the urine.

Treatment: Most patients will recover after some months, or even years. In some cases drugs, such as steroids, may be ordered. In a few cases tuberculosis supervenes, and the specific treatment for this will be ordered.

Sciatica

This is pain in the nerve which runs down the back of the thigh to the leg (Sciatic Nerve), and it often occurs with Lumbago, which is pain in the small of the back (the lumbar region). This is because the sciatic nerve comes out from the spinal cord between the bones of the spine in the lumbar region, and if there is disease or abnormality in the lumbar region, the sciatic nerve may also be affected.

Sciatica may be due to bone changes in the spine itself, caused by arthritis; new growths; or what is known as "slipped disc", or prolapsed lumbar disc.

Treatment: The treatment is to remove the cause, if possible, and so investigations are carried out, to find the cause. X-ray pictures are taken of the lumbar area.

Rest, and drugs to relieve the pain, together with the application of heat, are often ordered. When the pain has ceased to trouble the patient, massage and physiotherapy are usually of value. A support for the spine may be helpful for some patients.

Slipped Disc (see p. 78).

Stenosis

Contraction or narrowing of an opening or channel—so impeding the movements of the contents, e.g. Pyloric stenosis (p. 80).

MITRAL STENOSIS. When scar tissue is formed, as a result of inflammation, and narrows the channel between the left atrium and left ventricle in the heart, e.g. after acute rheumatism.

St. Vitus Dance or Chorea

Chorea is closely connected with Acute Rheumatism but nerve tissue is affected in Chorea, whilst in Acute Rheumatism it is the joints which are affected. The heart also may be involved. It occurs for the most part in children, mostly girls.

Symptoms: The child is restless and fidgets a great deal, and gives the impression of being clumsy. She may laugh or cry very easily, and often appears to be "making faces" and may be thought to be naughty or careless. It is at this stage that the real nature of the illness should be apparent, and treatment started immediately to prevent further progress of the disease and serious complications.

Chorea varies in degree from slight twitchings to violent jerky movements. The movements become worse if the child is excited, or knows that she is being watched.

Swallowing and speaking may become difficult, the appetite is variable, and there is severe loss of weight.

Treatment: Rest is most important to limit or prevent heart damage. The nurse must have patience and sympathy and a calm quiet manner to get the trust and confidence of the child.

Two nurses should move the child, to prevent her from exerting herself, and the same nurses should care for the child, whenever possible, so that the patient knows and trusts them. The nurses will also understand the child and note any change or development in the condition.

The child should be kept in bed, in a quiet room, or the bed screened, if in the ward. Cot sides may be necessary to prevent her from falling, and these should be padded. Penicillin is ordered.

Care of the skin is very important, because there is real danger of sores being caused by the friction and movements. Wool and bandages may be applied to protect parts, as necessary. A daily bath is given.

The Mouth must have routine care, and this may be difficult, because of the involuntary movements. Forceps should be avoided, as they may injure the delicate lining (mucous membrane) of the mouth.

Feeding is also difficult. Soft easily digested foods and plenty of fluids should be given, by the nurse, without haste. A feeding cup with a tube on the spout is useful. China and glass should not be used until the movements are controlled. In a very severe case, tube feeding may be used.

The temperature, pulse and respirations are taken and recorded, four-hourly, the thermometer being held carefully in the axilla or groin. The bowels should be opened regularly. The use of the bedpan creates problems, as the involuntary movements may cause it to be upset or spilled. The nurse should stay with the child, so helping to prevent an accident, but if a bedpan is upset the child must not be blamed, as she is already hypersensitive, and may become very disturbed.

A rubber bedpan is useful, otherwise padding may be applied to the ordinary bedpan.

If there is constipation a small enema of plain water may be given. Some kind of aspirin is ordered usually and a sedative at night to ensure rest and sleep.

The condition often improves in two or three weeks, and the physiotherapist then starts teaching the child simple exercises, before she is allowed to get up. Convalescence follows, before the child is allowed back to school.

Stroke (see p. 7).

T

Thyroid

The thyroid gland lies at the front of the neck, and secretes an important substance, the hormone known as thyroxin. This controls the activity of the body cells and the production of heat and energy in the body.

If the gland secretes too much of the hormone, the activity of the cells of the body is abnormally increased. This is known as hyperthyroidism, thyrotoxicosis, toxic goitre, exophthalmic goitre, or sometimes Graves's disease (from the name of Dr. Graves, who first described it). If the gland does not produce enough thyroxin the activity of the body becomes reduced and sluggish. This is known as hypothyroidism or myxoedema.

Hyperthyroidism is more common in women than men, and is often seen in quite young women. In many cases the gland is enlarged but *not* always. The enlargement is known as a goitre. In spite of having a good appetite and eating well, the patient loses weight, and is nervous restless, anxious and irritable and is unable to sleep well. She complains of feeling hot, of sweating profusely, and often that the bowels are opened more frequently than usual. In many cases, the eyes may be protruding, so that the patient appears to be staring, open-eyed. This is known as Exophthalmos, hence the description—exophthalmic goitre.

On admission to hospital, which will be some days before the operation the patient should be nursed in quiet surroundings. Visitors may be limited so that the patient is not over-excited or disturbed. It is important for the nurse to gain the confidence of the patient and to settle her fears as much as possible. A tactful nurse can be a great help in these cases. It is often helpful to introduce her, if possible, to a patient who has already had a similar condition and operation in order to encourage her and allay her fears.

The signs of heart complications must be watched for: e.g. breathlessness, oedema, etc. If these are noticed, or complained of, by the patient, they must be reported, and the doctor will order drugs for this.

The eyes may have to be protected with eye shields if there is a great deal of protrusion.

Drugs may be ordered to reduce the activity of the gland and improve the condition of the patient. (This may have been started some time previously, before admission to hospital).

Some surgeons do not allow any skin preparation to be done until the patient is in the theatre in order to avoid making her more nervous.

If the skin is to be prepared, it will be from the line of the chin above to the front of the chest wall over the sternum below.

At the operation, the surgeon removes a large amount of the gland, maybe as much as five-sixths.

Post-operatively: When the patient recovers from the effects of the anaesthetic she is propped up in bed, well supported with pillows, so that the neck is not stretched. The dressing on the wound should be specially protected if there is any vomiting. The pulse rate is counted every half hour at first, and charted separately. The usual 4 hourly temperature, pulse and respiration chart is kept. If the pulse rate rises it should be reported immediately and the temperature taken again. This may signify that too much thyroxin has entered the blood from the cut gland during the operation, a condition known as a *thyroid crisis* or acute thyrotoxicosis. With modern methods of surgery, it is now rare for this to be seen, but it must be watched for as immediate treatment is needed. It occurs in the first 24–48 hours after operation if it occurs at all.

To prevent this, fluids may be ordered and given intravenously, per rectum, or subcutaneously (under the skin), and iodine (as Potassium iodide) is given to block the over-production of the hormone. Large quantities of fluids are given by mouth when possible. Drugs, such as morphine, may be ordered to be given as required.

A HANDBOOK FOR NURSES

The dressing is watched for any signs of haemorrhage and reported upon if any undue bleeding seems to be taking place. Otherwise, the dressing is left for 24 hours and is then changed. If a drainage tube has been inserted, this is removed at the same time, unless there is a great amount of discharge from the wound. The clips or stitches are removed in the first 3 to 4 days in order to reduce the risk of an obvious scar. A dry dressing may be applied for a day or two, if the patient feels uncomfortable.

Diet: As soon as the patient can swallow confidently, a normal diet is given, but for the first few days fluids and a soft diet are often preferred.

After the first day, the patient will be allowed to sit out of bed, and should be encouraged to walk about as soon as possible.

GOITRE DUE TO IODINE LACK

Because the secretion of the thyroid gland contains a large amount of iodine, iodine is very important in the diet. It all comes, in the first place, from the sea. In some parts of the world, iodine may be lacking in the soil and the water supply, e.g., some parts of Derbyshire, Switzerland, New Zealand.

If the diet does not contain enough iodine, the thyroid gland will enlarge to try to overcome the deficiency. In some cases there is nothing else to be found, but a simple swelling, and the patient has no complaints. This is prevented now-a-days, by the addition of a minute amount of iodine to the diet, usually to the table salt, about 1 in 100,000 parts.

Later the swollen gland may cause trouble, by pressing on the trachea or the oesophagus, or may distress the patient by its appearance. In these cases, an operation is required.

Tonsil Abscess (Quinsy)

An abscess around the tonsil may be known as a Quinsy. There is great pain and there may be difficulty in both breathing and swallowing. The pain may be relieved by aspirin gargles. Nowadays antibiotics prevent this condition. The patient should be nursed sitting up so that if pus pours out if it can be expelled into a bowl or receiver immediately and not swallowed. If swallowing or breathing is difficult, and the abscess does not burst itself, it will be opened by the surgeon. A local anaesthetic is sprayed over the area and the quinsy is opened with a pair of quinsy forceps. The surgeon opens the forceps, when in position, so that the abscess is opened, and he then immediately withdraws them. The patient leans forward and expels the pus at once. If quinsy forceps are not to hand an ordinary scalpel may be used, after being prepared. This is done by wrapping adhesive strapping round the blade, leaving only the top half inch of the tip uncovered. This is then called a "guarded" scalpel. As soon as the abscess is opened, or bursts, the patient feels immediate relief. Gargles may be given frequently for a short time, to get rid of any further pus or blood which may escape from the area. Antibiotics may also be ordered by the doctor.

U

Ulcerative Colitis

The cause of an ulcerated large bowel (colon) is not understood, but the condition is most often seen in nervous, sensitive people, and it often starts in young people. The passage of blood and 'slime' with frequent diarrhoea causes severe illness. Medical treatment is successful in many cases, in keeping the patient well enough to lead a normal life, but there are often relapses. If the condition does not clear up under strict medical supervision, a surgeon may be asked to see if he considers that an operation would be advisable, to give the patient relief from the distressing condition. In some cases the deterioration of the patient is so rapid that an operation is urgently required. Surgical treatment is also indicated if the bowel perforates or becomes obstructed, or cancer occurs.

General treatment: Rest in bed, a good, nourishing diet, with very little roughage (or residue) are important. The meals must be made attractive, as the patient already has a poor appetite and is usually underweight.

Extra vitamins may be ordered, and a blood transfusion may be given if there is anaemia. Sulphonamides may be ordered.

Drinks should be given warm or cool, not hot or cold as these would stimulate the bowel to act. Such things as pre-digested foods may be given (Complan, Bengers) to increase the value of the diet. Antibiotics and cortisone drugs may be ordered by the doctor. Tincture of belladonna or of opium give relief to some cases, and these may be ordered. Antibiotics may be tried whilst the temperature is raised.

The frequent use of the bedpan will make it desirable to have the patient in a bed near to the sluice or toilet annexe. The side ward may be used, but the patient needs company and interest to keep her mind occupied and therefore she is often nursed in the general ward. Occupational therapy and a good library service are of value.

The number and kind of stools must be reported, and if a specimen is asked for it must be taken from a fresh stool.

The patient must be weighed each week and a record kept.

Operations. (1) *Ileostomy:* The ileum, (the last part of the small intestine, before it joins the large intestine) is brought to the surface of the abdomen, and opened, so that the faeces can pass through the opening. The part of the bowel which is ulcerated can therefore be rested and allowed to heal. If blood and mucus continue to be discharged, it may be necessary to remove the large bowel (colectomy).

(2) *Colectomy.* This is the name given to the operation for the removal of the large bowel. It may be done in two stages, the rectum being left, until later. If only half of the colon is removed, the operation is known as hemicolectomy, ('hemi'—before a word means half).

Before any of these operations, the preparation of the patient is important, because the patient's condition is not good. Drugs will be ordered to reduce the amount of infection in the bowel. A light diet is given, with a low residue (to avoid stimulating the bowel) such things as soup, custard, strained fruit juices, milk puddings forming the basis. Intravenous fluids and blood transfusions may be ordered to improve the general condition.

Post-operatively: When the patient recovers from the anaesthetic, he is nursed in an upright position, well supported and comfortable. Intravenous fluids are usually continued, and a fluid intake and output chart is kept. Fluids are given by mouth, when the patient is ready for these, but no solid food for at least the first two days. Then a light diet is introduced and gradually increased. Drugs will be continued for a few days to prevent infection. Vitamins may be ordered, and if the discharge from the opening is very fluid, substances such as Isogel may be given. The dressing on the wound will need to be changed daily, and the stitches may be removed on the 8th or 10th day. A special bag (ileostomy bag) is fitted over the artificial opening to prevent the intestinal contents from coming in contact with the skin, as this would irritate it and make it sore. The bag is of light polythene, and has a substance around its opening which makes it stick to the skin, and which also protects the skin. The bag also collects the discharge from the opening, which can be renewed as necessary or emptied, washed and replaced. Several types of these bags are available.

A special association has been formed for people who have an ileostomy (the Ileostomy Association). The patient should be put in touch with the association through the medical social worker. By joining the association the patient receives all the advice and encouragement needed to live a normal active life.

Ulcers

An ulcer is a breakdown of any surface of the body where the cells die and are cast off as a slough (pronounced 'sluff') leaving a raw area. For example there may be ulcers of the skin, ulcers of the mouth, the tongue, the stomach, the intestines, the rectum, and ulcers of the bladder.

Ulcers may be due to: (a) lack of circulation to the part, such as in bedsores, (b) injury, where the wound has become infected and the bacteria prevent healing taking place, (c) chemicals, such as acids, (d) certain diseases such as tuberculosis, (e) heat or cold, which may destroy the surface cells, (f) nervous conditions, where the nerve supply to the part is defective, or (g) they may arise from some unknown cause and they are often associated with anxiety.

GASTRIC AND DUODENAL ULCERS—**Peptic**

Ulcers in the lining of the stomach and duodenum (the first part of the intestine) are common, and, if medical treatment fails to cure the condition operation is often required. These two are classed together as *Peptic Ulcers*.

GASTRIC ULCER

This is seen more often in men than in women, and usually between the ages of 35 and 55 years. It usually occurs in men who have irregular meals, because of their work, or who are prone to worry and anxiety. The patient complains of vague attacks of "indigestion" for some months. Later the following symptoms occur:

Pain is felt in the region of the stomach (*epigastric pain*) soon after a meal, and this may be followed by vomiting, which relieves the pain. There may be loss of weight, because the patient is disinclined to eat for fear of vomiting. If the ulcer breaks into a blood vessel in the wall of the stomach vomiting of blood may occur, known as *haematemesis*. This vomited blood may appear as a dark brown sediment because it has been acted upon by the gastric juices, and partly digested ('coffee grounds' in appearance). If there is a large amount of blood, it will look like blood, often in large dark-coloured clots, so that it appears almost like pieces of liver. This happens when a large blood vessel has been eroded by the ulcer, and the gastric juices have not been able to act on it before it is vomited. If a large amount of blood is vomited, and the bleeding does not stop, an emergency operation is often necessary.

Investigations are carried out; (a) *Barium meal* X-rays. The barium is given to the patient in a drink, which he swallows whilst standing in front of the X-ray viewing machine. As barium shows up on X-rays, the shape of the stomach and duodenum can be seen, and any abnormality caused by an ulcer (a crater) will be seen. (b) *Test Meals.* Substances are usually given by injection (e.g. histamine, insulin or pentagastrin) to stimulate the production of acid by the stomach. A gastric tube (e.g. Ryle's) is swallowed, the test substance is administered and samples of gastric juices are withdrawn with a syringe at regular stated intervals. The samples are placed in correctly labelled tubes and sent to the laboratory together with the request form. Here they are tested for the amount of acid and the presence of blood and bile. A patient with a duodenal ulcer will probably be producing large amounts of concentrated acid, while in the case of a cancerous ulcer of the stomach the acid will be weak or entirely absent.

(c) *Gastroscopy:* This is usually carried out in the morning, the patient not having had any food after an early supper on the previous evening. In preparation, the surgeon orders a sedative to be given. The procedure may be carried out with a local anaesthetic, the patient being given anaesthetic tablets to suck beforehand.

A tube with a flexible end containing an electric light and an arrangement of small lenses, is passed through the mouth into the stomach. This is the gastroscope, and through it the surgeon is able to see the inside of the stomach. No food is allowed after this has been carried out for at least 2 or 3 hours, until the effect of the anaesthetic has passed off. This is because there will be lack of feeling in the parts affected by the anaesthetic, and food or drink may be inhaled instead of swallowed, or the patient may scald himself with hot fluids.

(d) *Test for Occult Blood:* In cases where an ulcer is suspected, but there is no visible bleeding, a specimen of the stool (faeces) may be asked for, and this is collected and sent to the laboratory. Tests carried out to find if there is any unseen (occult) blood present. When this test is to be carried out, special instructions regarding the diet will be given. Some foods, such as meat and fish may be forbidden for two days before the specimens are to be collected. The reason for this is that some foods contain the same substances as human blood, and may give an incorrect result if they are present in the specimen.

Treatment: Bed rest, diet and drugs are part of the treatment given in cases of gastric ulcer, before operation is decided upon. The drugs are given to reduce the acidity of the stomach contents, and are known as antacids. Many ulcers will heal after a few weeks of this regime. If not, or if there is a relapse after healing has taken place, an operation is advised.

DUODENAL ULCER

The differences between a gastric and a duodenal ulcer are mainly in the signs and symptoms. If the ulcer is in the duodenum, the pain will be felt $1\frac{1}{2}$ to 3 hours after taking a meal, and is often described as hunger pain, because the patient is relieved by taking food. The pain may waken the patient during the night, so he may get into the habit of taking some food during the night. Vomiting is not common, but blood may be passed in the stools. If there is a large amount of blood, escaping from the ulcer the stools look very dark coloured, and "tarry". This is known as *Melaena*. The *treatment* for a duodenal ulcer is rather similar to that for a gastric ulcer, rest and diet and antacids are advised, but if the ulcer continues to trouble the patient and prevent him from working an operation is performed.

OPERATIONS FOR DUODENAL AND GASTRIC ULCERS

1. *Partial Gastrectomy.* The lower end of the stomach is removed, and the remaining part is stitched either to the duodenum or to the intestine.

2. *Vagotomy:* The nerves (Vagus nerves) which supply the stomach are part of the Autonomic Nervous System which is not controlled by the brain. In vagotomy, the surgeon cuts the vagus nerves, which results in less activity of the muscles in the wall of the stomach, and there is also a decrease in the amount of acid secreted. Vagotomy is usually carried out with either a gastroenterostomy (see below) or a plastic operation on the pylorus (pyloroplasty).

3. *Gastro-enterostomy:* A new opening is made between the stomach and intestine so that the food does not have to pass through the pyloric end of the stomach, where ulcers are most likely to occur.

4. *Antrectomy.* The pyloric end of the stomach only is removed as this is the part concerned with the secretion of acid.

5. *Total Gastrectomy* is a very severe operation and may be carried out for carcinoma of the stomach, when the whole organ is removed. This leaves the patient without a reservoir for food, and is not often performed. After the stomach has been removed the oesophagus is joined (anastomosed) to the intestine, so that food passes through the tract without gastric digestion.

POST-OPERATIVE CARE. Intravenous blood or fluids will be given in most cases. The patient is sat up in bed as soon as possible, well supported with pillows. The care of the mouth is very important, as he will not be allowed any solid food for some days. A special diet is ordered of fluids only, for the first 4 or 5 days. The contents of the stomach are aspirated back through a naso-gastric tube at intervals for the following two or three days. A chart of the fluid intake and output is maintained, and when the amount of gastric fluid aspirated falls to 30 ml the surgeon will probably order that the naso-gastric tube be removed. Drugs may be ordered for the relief of pain, and to ensure rest at night. The pressure areas will require frequent attention. The pulse rate will be taken regularly and charted accurately. A flatus tube may be passed to relieve any distension, but an enema or suppository may be ordered for the 4th or 5th day. If there is a drainage tube in the wound, any discharge must be reported, otherwise it is removed, usually on the 2nd or 3rd day. Stitches are removed on the 8th to 10th day, and deep sutures, if these have been used, will remain until the 14th or 15th day after operation.

On leaving hospital, the patient is advised as to his diet, the need for rest, and the temporary avoidance of alcohol and irritating foods, such as spices, mustard, etc. A normal diet should be possible after a few weeks. It is important that the patient should avoid anxiety and worry and, if his work is a source of worry or distress, he would be advised to try to find less upsetting work.

Undescended Testicle

The testicles (or testes) are glands which develop near the kidneys before birth, but, at birth both should be in the scrotum, which is a pouch of soft tissue and skin. They are not able to function normally if they do not descend, and there is also danger of malignancy. An undescended testicle is often associated with a hernia.

Treatment: An operation is carried out at about 4–5 years of age. Usually the testicle is brought down and placed in the scrotum and secured in the correct position by the surgeon. Special instructions will be given to the nurse about the post-operative care, and the removal of any special stitch or retaining apparatus.

Uraemia

This is the name given to the condition when the kidneys fail to carry out their functions. The substances, which should be excreted in the urine, are held in the body, and they accumulate in the blood, because the kidneys are not working properly. Another name for this condition is Chronic Renal Failure.

The substances which should be excreted are toxic, i.e., poisonous to the body, and are the waste products of combustion, that is, the waste produced by the using up of the food in the body. When these waste substances are circulating in the blood, they reach and affect all the systems of the body.

Urine: The Specific Gravity of the urine remains stationary around 1010 to 1015. The urine contains albumen and parts of the lining of the kidney tubes (casts). The patient's sleep may be disturbed by having to pass urine during the night.

Skin: This becomes dry and yellowish in colour. There may be great irritation and itching (pruritis) as the sweat glands are excreting some of the substances usually excreted by the kidneys.

Circulatory System: There is always some anaemia. This system is affected by the hypertension (High Blood Pressure) which is always present and not by the failure of the kidneys. The patient may have a stroke, others die from heart failure.

Digestive System: The breath may smell of urine. The tongue is dry, dirty, brown, and coated. There may be a feeling of sickness, (nausea) or actual vomiting, and there may be diarrhoea. Hiccups commonly occurs, and causes the patient great discomfort.

Respiratory System: The breathing becomes deeper, as the waste in the body circulates in the blood, and the lungs try to expel some of it.

Nervous System: The patient complains of feeling tired, at first, but then becomes drowsy, and later goes into a coma (deep unconsciousness). Fits, with muscular twitchings, like epilepsy, may occur in the later stages.

Treatment: The diet may be restricted to a low protein diet, (mainly of carbohydrates and fat, but with very little meat, fish, fowl, eggs, cheese, etc.) and extra fluids are given, and, in some cases, extra salt to make up for what is being lost.

However, as nothing can be done to improve or cure the condition, some doctors allow the patient to have whatever he fancies. A blood transfusion may be given slowly for the anaemia, and certain drugs may be ordered to reduce the blood pressure.

V

Varicose Veins

A varicose vein is a vein which is tortuous (twisted) and enlarged (dilated). The valves in the vein do not function normally, so that blood does not flow back to the heart and will tend to stagnate.

Haemorrhoids have already been described, and these are varicose veins of the rectum.

Varicose Veins of the Legs. The common site for varicose veins is in the legs, particularly in women. They may be caused by:

(a) Weakness of the walls or valves of the veins. Such a weakness may run in families (it is inherited).

(b) Long periods of standing, when the return of the blood is more difficult. Normally the action of the leg muscles on walking is to massage the blood back to the heart. On standing, stagnation of blood is liable to occur.

(c) Any obstruction to the venous return of the blood, such as garters, or by tumours in the pelvis and abdomen.

(d) They may occur in a pregnant woman, due to the weight of the baby and the pressure in the abdomen on the veins. If the woman already suffers from varicose veins, they may become worse during pregnancy.

Signs and Symptoms: The patient may complain of aching and tiredness after a period of standing. The ankles may become swollen, especially in the later part of the day. The veins will stand out, and become unsightly, this often being the reason why the patient seeks the doctor's advice.

Treatment: If seen in the early stages, the application of an elastic bandage or an elastic stocking may be sufficient, by giving support.

Injections: The surgeon may inject into the vein a solution which will cause that area of vein to close up and become fibrous. The blood from the part below is able to return through other vessels, as they all branch and intermingle. This method of treatment is only satisfactory for small surface vessels.

Ligatures: The vein, which is usually the long saphenous vein in the leg, may be tied off with ligatures at the top, in the groin, where it joins the femoral vein. Ligatures are also placed above and below the knee, and at the ankle. With this treatment, injections may also be given.

Stripping: In this case, the vein is also ligatured in the groin, and a special instrument known as a stripper is passed inside the length of the vessel, and withdrawn through the tissues, so as to completely remove the vein. As this is being done, the leg is bandaged firmly with a crepe bandage from the toes upwards, and any hollows may be filled with pads of felt. This pressure prevents excess oozing of blood and bruising. Some bruising is often seen after the operation, and the nurse should reassure the patient that this will soon clear up. The incisions in the groin and at the ankle are stitched, and the stitches removed in 7 to 14 days, according to the surgeon's instructions.

The patient is encouraged to get up and walk about the day after the operation in order to encourage the circulation through the other vessels. *Complications* which may follow varicose veins are:

(*a*) *Rupture:* This means that the vein breaks, in which case there is need for immediate treatment, as a great amount of blood may be lost in a very short time, and may cause death. The *first aid treatment* is to lie the patient down, raise the limb, and apply pressure to the bleeding point, firmly, until a doctor is available, or the patient is taken to hospital. A tourniquet should *not* be applied.

(*b*) *Phlebitis:* This is inflammation of the vein and the formation of a clot in the vein (thrombophlebitis). This causes pain, and soothing dressings may be applied, such as lead and opium lotion, or kaolin. Drugs may be ordered in case of infection.

(*c*) *Varicose Ulcers:* These may develop in a chronic case. After some slight injury, such as a knock, the skin of the leg becomes hard, dry and discoloured, and finally breaks down. Open sores result which may be very persistent, and these are then known as Varicose Ulcers. Because these ulcers are partly due to the blood tending to drop to the lower part of the body by gravity (as any fluid or article always falls down, towards the earth) they are sometimes called Gravitational Ulcers.

The Treatment of Varicose Ulcers: Conservative treatment is tried first, in almost all cases.

This may be:

(*a*) rest in bed, with the foot of the bed elevated, so that the heart is on a lower level than the feet, and the blood drains back more easily, so emptying the veins and allowing healing to take place.

(*b*) strong support with elastic bandages combined with massage and exercises. This is to encourage the use of the muscles of the legs, for they squeeze the veins and help pump the blood up towards the heart.

(*c*) Operation. The vein may have to be ligated, as already described. The ulcer area is cut away (excised) and a skin graft may be applied to the part a few days later.

INDEX

Abscess 1
—Appendix 8
—Brain 12
—Pelvic 8
—Subphrenic 8
—Tonsil 90
Acute Rheumatism 83
Adenitis 2
Amnesia 2
Amputation 2
Anaemia 3
Anal Fissure 4
Anal Fistula 5
Anaphylaxis 5
Aneurysm 6
Apoplexy 7
Appendicitis 8
Appendicectomy 8
Appendix Abscess 8
Arteriosclerosis 9
Arthritis 9
Arthrodesis 11
Arthroplasty 11
Ascites 11
Atheroma 11

Blood Pressure 42
Boils 12
Brain Abscess 12
—Haemorrhage 7
Bright's Disease 68
Burns and Scalds 12
Bronchitis Acute 13
—Chronic 14
Bronchiectasis 14
Bronchopneumonia 15
Bronchial Carcinoma 16
Buerger's Disease 16

Cancer (Carcinoma) 17
Carbuncle 18
Cerebral Compression 18
Cholecystitis 19
Cholecystectomy 20

Cholecystotomy 20
Choledocotomy 20
Chorea 86
Colles Fracture 21
Colostomy 22
Coma 23
Concussion 23
Coronary Thrombosis 42
Chron's Disease 23
Cross Infection 24
Constipation 24
Cystitis 25
Cystoscopy 26

Diabetes 27
Diabetic Coma 28
Diarrhoea 29
Disseminated Sclerosis 30
Duodenal Ulcer 93
Dyspepsia 31
Dysphagia 31

Embolus 32
Empyema 61
Epilepsy (Fits) 33

Fractures 34

Gangrene 36
Gastric Ulcer 93
Gastritis 37

Haemorrhoids 38
Haemothorax 39
Heart Disease 40
Hernia 43
Hodgkin's Disease 46
Hydrocele 46
Hysteria 46

Incontinence 47
Infectious Diseases 48
Infective Hepatitis 55
Insulin 27
Intestinal Obstruction 56
Intussusception 57

Jaundice 58

Kidney Operations 58

Leukaemia 60
Lung Operations 61
Lymphoma 63

Mastectomy 64
Meningitis 66
Migraine 67
Myxoedema 67

Nephritis 68

Oedema 70

Paralysis 71
Paralytic Ileus 72
Peritonitis 8
Phimosis 73
Phlebitis 99
Piles 38
Pilonidal Sinus 74
Pneumoconiosis 74
Pneumonia 75
Pneumothorax 75

Post-menopausal bleeding 17
Prostatectomy 76
Protrusion of Disc 78
Purpura 79
Pyelitis 79
Pyloric Stenosis 80

Raynaud's Disease 82
Retrograde Amnesia 2
Rheumatism 83
Rib Fracture 84
Rigor 85
Rupture 43

Sarcoidosis 85
Scalds 12
Sciatica 86
Slipped Disc 78
Stenosis 86
St. Vitus Dance 86
Stroke 7
Sympathectomy 16

Thyroid 88
Tonsil Abscess 90

Ulcerative Colitis 91
Ulcers 93
Under water seal 76
Undescended Testicle 96
Uraemia 97

Varicose Veins 98
Volvulus 57

X-Rays 20, 25, 64, 77, 94